HUGS FROM THE REFRIGERATOR

James McClernan, Ed.D.

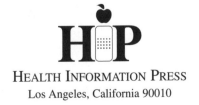

HEALTH INFORMATION PRESS
Los Angeles, California 90010

Library of Congress Cataloging-in-Publication Data

McClernan, James 1935-
   Hugs from the refrigerator: the psychology of emotional eating / James
   McClernan.
      p. cm.
   Previously published: Kansas City, Mo.: Westport Publishers, 1994.
   Includes index.
   ISBN 1-885987-21-8
   1. Weight loss. I. Title.

RM222.2 .M4334 2000
613.7'1--dc21   00-059691

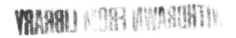

DISCLAIMER
The information presented in this book is based on the experience and interpretation
of the author. Although the information has been carefully researched and checked
for accuracy, currency and completeness, neither the author nor the publisher accept
any responsibility or liability with regard to errors, omissions, misuse or misinter-
pretation.

ISBN: 1-885987-21-8
Printed in the United States of America

Health Information Press
4727 Wilshire Blvd., Suite 300
Los Angeles, CA 90010
1-800-MED-SHOP
Internet: HIPBOOKS.COM

TABLE OF CONTENTS

PREFACE

Since his last book, Change Your Mind: Change Your Weight (Health Plus Publishers, 1985), Dr. James McClernan has a much expanded story to tell and a beautiful new way to tell it. Although his earlier convictions about the subject of weight loss hold firm, his depth of understanding is greater and his insights into the possibilities for human change and long-term success are clearer and stronger.

The purpose of this book is two-fold:

1. To facilitate readers in the development of the personal self-efficacy necessary for the self-directed, successful, long-term weight loss; and

2. To expose, through extensive research and documentation, commercial weight loss programs and products; why they don't work; how they damage health, waste money, and in fact detract from their goal.

In 1990, the nation's 33 billion dollar fat industry earned a congressional investigation. In 1998, it merited a Federal Trade Commission (FTC) review. Although some weight loss products have improved in content and/or moved under the so-called "protective" eye of financially-strapped hospitals, the flow of new drugs promoting weight loss has proven to be dangerous. The odds for long-term, successful weight loss have certainly not improved in recent years—in fact, they may even have gotten worse.

It is believed that only 5 percent of dieters experience long-term weight loss success (i.e., weight loss that is maintained for 30 months or more after leaving a weight loss program)—meaning that a shocking 95 percent of dieters regain their lost pounds, or even more.[1-4] Even though new studies by the National Weight Loss Registry provide some signs of hope for long-term dieters, the point is that the vast majority of dieters are unable to maintain their weight loss in the long term.[5] Such consumers end up feeling disillusioned, angry, depressed, hopeless, and helpless. This may put them in a weakened state of health and make them even more vulnerable to additional weight gain. Certainly it leaves them with a good deal less money in their pockets for having made an effort to lose weight.

While the bad news is that commercial weight loss programs do not work—and can be dangerous to your health as well; the good news is that there is a means by which any individual can successfully lose excess weight and keep it off, permanently and healthfully, without financial ruin. The solution is simple, but must be earned through desire and the willingness to risk changing not only one's behavior, but also one's self-image that has contributed to being overweight. This is achieved after learning to follow and love a self-empowerment process that builds self-efficacy, that encourages mastery of a discipline (such as tai chi, yoga or meditation), and that promotes a wellness lifestyle.

Hugs from the Refrigerator: The Psychology of Emotional Eating emphasizes developing a preference for and deriving pleasure from healthful eating and sensible exercise as a means of achieving and maintaining ideal weight. "Gradual" is a key word in Dr. McClernan's "System for Healthful Eating" (S.H.E.) and his program of "Healthful Exercise" (H.E.). These systems eliminate the structured "control" dieters may subconsciously rebel against and encourage the development of a self-designed program on a long-term basis. By using expanded self-awareness and perspectives, lowered expectations, and balanced attitudes; and by staying on the edge of their comfort zone and giving themselves permission to change, individuals can and do make meaningful shifts.

Hugs from the Refrigerator addresses such major considerations as how to stop procrastinating, how to move from relying on external motivations to understanding how to develop self-motivation, and how to stop sabotaging behaviors. All of these factors are vital to long-term success and offer much more hope than do weight loss gimmicks.

Dr. McClernan guides readers to an understanding of the underlying causes of their problems. He illustrates many common dilemmas with the story of Louise, who Dr. McClernan has counseled, and who is representative of the many clients he has nurtured on their way to finding their own truths. Together, Dr. McClernan and Louise inspire readers to embark on their own adventure and encourage them to confront the pain and fear holding them back so that they are able to find their own answers.

Dr. McClernan realizes that just as there is no single cause of obesity, there is no single cure for it, either. He is gently sensitive to the health and social problems the chronically overweight person encounters. He is empathetic to what it is like to carry the burden of excess weight in a world that lauds the trim and denigrates the obese.

How a person feels and what is experienced in one's life have everything to do with how many "hugs from the refrigerator" seem necessary. The facts that 85 percent of the people participating in weight loss programs are perfectionists and that 90 percent or more are eating in response to their feelings, are dramatically presented through one composite story—a story that includes the struggles that almost every one of us goes through with our parents, siblings, education, career, and families, only not always with the omnipresent handicap and additional burden of being overweight.

Genetic circumstances and behavioral conditioning are addressed in this book, but only as inhibitors to weight loss, not as conditions that preclude weight loss. The primary focus of this book, Louise's story, as well as the author's professional, practical how-to summaries, lead to the understanding that chronic undesirable weight cycles can be broken and a desired lifestyle established which will bring rewards far beyond a permanent healthful and attractive weight.

REFERENCES

1. Warshaw R: "Fat Chance." *Philadelphia Inquirer*, Mar 8, 1992, p. 26+.

2. "Dieting, Weight Loss Myths, Blasted." *Psychology Today*, Mar/Apr 2000, p. 20.

3. Syngal S, et al.: "Long-Term Weight Patterns and Risk for Cholecystectomy in Women." *Annals of Internal Medicine* 1999; 130(6): 471-477.

4. French SA et al.: "Weight Variability and Incident Diseasein Older Women: the Iowa Women's Health Study." *International Journal of Obesity and Related Metabolic Disorders*, Mar 1997; 21(3): 217-223.

5. Polivy J: "The Mythology of Dieting." *Healthy Weight Journal*, Jan/Feb 1999; 13(1). Available online at: *http://www.healthyweightnetwork.com/editor.htm*, 9/22/00.

Introduction

"YES, BUT WILL I KEEP IT OFF?"

L *ate in the evening, while driving home from yet another weight loss* support group, my thoughts about the ever-burgeoning fat industry keep drifting. First, to the sad realization that commercial weight loss organizations and product manufacturers reap great financial profits while individual success with long-term weight loss is dismally low, and then to the recent alarms that there is a global epidemic of obesity, especially among young people.[1-5] After years of yelling into the wind, I'm starting to see a ground swell of concern by American and international health care organizations as the number of obesity-related illnesses and resulting deaths continues to mount. Health care professionals are no longer indifferent to the facts and, along with overweight consumers, they are now seeking something other than magic illusions as an easy escape from some difficult questions. Obesity is now second only to smoking as the leading preventable cause of death in the world.[6]

I reflect, too, on the more meaningful, probing questions people are asking as they look for facts and substance in the easy promises thrown at them. At the same time, I note the increasing numbers of people joining the fast weight-loss industry as it continues to grow annually—from a $33 billion industry in 1995 to a $50 billion industry in 2000.[7] Even though there is plenty of published research showing that diets lead to added pounds, in their desperation, consumers continue to purchase an endless flow of diet books and programs. The search for something better is more urgent than ever. And although the new weight loss products and services have new names, they rely on the same old recycled magic.

My hope is that in this time of quantum world changes and a plentiful international economy, more people will be able to eat better, and we can concentrate on repairing some of the damage we have done to our environment—and maybe we will also be ready to take responsibility for repairing our bodies by using our minds, and finding a new belief in ourselves.

As I climb into bed, my spirits are up and I slip into a hope-filled vision of a new social movement as powerful and more rapid than the quit-smoking trends: a time when well-being and wellness are the norm.

When I awaken the next morning, the revealing light of the new day raises new questions in my mind. In this throw-away world of plenty, where so many of us are dependent on high technology, addicted to quick fixes, and stressed because of time crunches, nomadic job changes, and the uncertainty of corporate mergers, is the idea of a self-correcting activity "marketable"? We always are led to believe that the next answer is just around the corner: artificial sweeteners, low- or non-fat foods, and pills that burn fat off while we sleep—these are promises from which it is difficult to distract the longing consumer. Will the overweight person choose to pursue a better quality, healthy life? Are the overweight ready to buy into real change? Is it the right time to find the magic inside of us?

We seem to have no new answers for the obesity epidemic. The promise for the future seems to be found in the latest medication that looks good in animal testing. Although we now know more about our genes and the processes of the brain that trigger eating, we have no more real answers than we did decades ago. Even the developing countries, where food was hard to come by, there is a rising prevalence of major obesity-related health problems, now that more food is available.[8,9] However, is it only the result of greater availability of food, or does it belie a much more complex problem?

Just as I have taken the time to survey people who have been able to lose the extra pounds and keep them off, so have several other university researchers. Even though these individuals may reflect only a small percentage of our international weight loss concerns, they hold the important answers that are unavailable in the commercial weight loss industry. These successful people who have kept their unwanted pounds off for five years or more are not hard to find and have provided us with new insights that are relatively consistent. The studies I completed prior to 1995 and the research currently being done look at thousands of individuals who have kept the weight off. The answers to how they did so have their base in what is happening inside the individual, and not on some external magic. The new question, then, is to determine how the *internal* magic button can be turned on.

The heroine of this book, Louise, is in the process of becoming what she has so long been distracted from—the woman she believes in. In her journey, her extra fat is removed in a way no weight loss program can ever account for—i.e., by an intrinsic power that can come only from the heart of each individual. Maybe the next hero or heroine is you!

Please leave any preconceived ideas aside when you read this book. Open the book, and open your mind. Move through the pages and allow yourself to discover the core of your power. Go beyond your dreams and illusions, beyond your fears and the limitations you've put on yourself. Expect to go much further than just being permanently trim. Expect the unending excitement of discovering all the best inside you.

Let this story be yours. New horizons, a new life, a new world: all created by you.

REFERENCES

1. Fine JT, et al. "A Prospective Study of Weight Change and Health-Related Quality of Life in Women." *JAMA*, Dec 8 1999; 282(22): 2136-2142.

2. Mokdad AH, et al. "The Spread of the Obesity Epidemic in the United States, 1991-1998." *JAMA*, Oct 27 1999; 292(15): 1519-1522.

3. "Patient Page: Weight Management." *JAMA*, Oct 27 1999; 292(15): 1596.

4. Kopelman PG: "Obesity as a Medical Problem." *Nature*, Apr 6, 2000; 404(6778): 634-643.

5. Reuters America, Inc. "Obesity an Epidemic—Among Kids, Too—U.S. Conference." Washington, DC; dateline Oct 19, 1998.

6. Hunter SM, et al. "Roles of Mental Health Professionals in Multidisciplinary Medically Supervised Treatment Programs for Obesity." *Southern Medical Journal*, Jun 1997; 90(6): 578-586.

7. Friedman JM: "Obesity in the New Millennium." *Nature*, Apr 6, 2000; 404(6778): 632-634.

8. Marchessault G, et al.: "WA Global Approach to Obesity." *Healthy Weight Journal*, Nov/Dec 1999; 13(6). Available online at: *http://www.healthyweightnetwork.com/editor.htm*, 9/22/00.

9. World Health Organization Conference, "Consultation on Obesity." Geneva, Jun 3-5, 1997; "Prevention and Management of Obesity," Tokyo, Dec. 1998. Press release for 1997 available online at: *http://www.who-int/archives/inf-pr-1997/en/pr97-46.html*, 9/25/00.

Prologue

THE GREAT FAT
RIP-OFFS

A *ccording to the 1988 report issued by Surgeon General C. Everett* Koop, diet-related diseases accounted for 68 percent of all deaths in the U.S.[1] In 1995, the total cost spent as a result of obesity amounted to $99.2 billion dollars. Approximately 51.6 billion of those dollars were direct medical costs.[2] In 1998, Dr. David Satcher, the present Surgeon General and former head of the Centers for Disease Control and Prevention, indicated we spend only 1 percent of our budget on prevention.[3]

Americans now spend $50 billion every year trying to lose weight.[4] A survey by the U.S. Government indicates that half of all American women and one-quarter of all American men are on a diet at any given moment. We buy diet pills, exercise equipment, liquid diets, packaged foods, and diet books. We join weight loss groups, exercise centers, and hospital-sponsored weight loss programs. We submit to hypnosis and liposuction, we have our stomachs stapled and our jaws wired... yet more than 95 percent of us who try one or more of these weight loss methods either fail to lose any significant amount of weight, or we regain it within a short period of time. That the international girth continues to grow is clearly demonstrated by the fact that manufacturers of public seating (i.e., airlines, theaters, sports stadiums) are having to expand the size of the seats. The weight loss industry pledges to help, yet, at their best, weight loss programs "produce and maintain only about a ten percent reduction in body weight for about a year," says the North American Association for the Study of Obesity released in February, 1999. After two investigative studies and conferences (1990 and

1998), The Federal Trade Commission (FTC) finally issued new "voluntary" guidelines,[5] a tiny step aimed at giving consumers more information about the huge numbers of largely unregulated diet programs across the country.

THE LONG-TERM SUCCESS AND SAFETY OF DIET PROGRAMS AND PRODUCTS

The commercial weight loss industry has published little or no follow-up studies of a long-term nature. The 1998 FTC report disclosed that none of the five leading weight loss companies offers any reliable information about their success rates—nor have they allowed objective researchers to evaluate them.[6] One smaller company, The Diet Workshop, estimates that only 7 to 8 percent of its customers reach their weight loss goal and maintain it for at least six months. The 1991 report indicated the Federal Trade Commission investigated more than a dozen diet programs and clinics that overstated their claims. Some of the larger programs pay university professors or private institutes to do research studies, but as soon as the research is paid for, it is under the control of the purchaser, who is free to decide just what the public will see. Being objective under these circumstances is extremely difficult.

Some commercial programs conduct no follow-up studies at all. They avoid questions about research by substituting dramatic examples or testimonials of consumers who have lost weight using their methods. These companies are also good at casting the blame for failures back on the individual, claiming that "people are not norms" (i.e., statistics do not determine individual behavior) or that the participants "did not follow the program as instructed." Additionally, because old programs and products peter out and new ones are born almost monthly, many companies can evade the question of documented, long-term successes by simply stating that, "it is too soon to tell," while implying that they have every reason to believe there will be a significant long-term success rate. Because we're eager to believe in the possibility of success, most of us are unlikely to press the issue any further.

One thing you can be absolutely sure of: if any weight loss method should be proven through independent, sound, indisputable and reproducible research to be safe and long-term effective for large numbers of people, you will read about it in the headlines.

However, the fact is, even though a great deal of sound and independent research on obesity—with a current annual price tag of $100 million[2]—has been conducted on an on-going basis for the past fifty years, little is known about the short- or long-term safety and effectiveness of most of the weight loss products and methods in use today. At this point, it appears as though no known program, plan, treatment, or product offers long-term effectiveness to other than a very small percentage of individuals. Because a certain number of individuals are going to be successful no matter which means or methods they chose to use to lose weight, it is very possible that the program or treatment involved cannot claim responsibility for even these few successes. There's even indication that the programs may be contributing to the problem.

Here are just a few examples from the massive amount of research literature that will give you more than sufficient cause to exercise caution before using any commercial program, product, or treatment for weight loss:

- Even though diet drugs have proven to be dismal failures, the marketing is more aggressive and sales have shot from $37.7 billion in 1990 to $78.9 billion in 1997. A new study in the *Journal of the American Medical Association* shows that obese volunteers taking Orlistat, a drug that blocks absorption of about 30 percent of the fat in foods, lost an average of 19 pounds, as compared to a 13 pound weight loss in a placebo group.[7] The safety of Orlistat remains in doubt. A previous study found 12 cases of breast cancer among 1,063 women taking the drug.[8]

- The first wrongful-death suit against the manufacture of fen-phen (fenfluramine-phentermine) used in combination with Redux, was settled for an undisclosed amount.[9] It was one of 3,200 lawsuits pending against the pharmaceutical giant American Home Products Corporation.

- The Federal Trade Commission sued SlimAmerica, Inc., for deceptive advertising in newspapers, on the Internet, and in magazines such as the *Ladies Home Journal* and *Cosmopolitan.* A U.S. District Court in Florida found that the company had made false claims about its diet products, which were billed as a "New Triple Medical Breakthrough," and ordered $8 million paid in redress.[10] Other medications such as Ephedrine and even some herbal products such as Cellasene have recently been taken of the market. Yet even while some oral weight loss products are being discontinued, at the same time new ones are taking their place.

- A survey of participants in a plan that used pre-packaged food and who elected to have their pictures and testimonials used in advertisements found that after only 20 months, all but 28 percent had regained their weight.[11]

- Patients treated surgically, through colon resectioning, stomach stapling, and balloon insertions, were all unsuccessful over the long term.[12] Surgical treatment, fasting, and behavior modification are equally unsuccessful after four years.[13]

- In one study, after four to five years following completion of a weight loss program, less than three percent of all subjects were at or below their post-treatment weight.[14]

- Dr. John Forest, Director of Nutrition Research at Baylor College of Medicine in Houston, completed a two-year study of 150 dieters. The conclusion? "Ninety-five percent of people who lose 40 pounds or more regain it in two years."[15]

- People who lose weight rapidly via fasting are up to three times as likely to gain it back as those who shed pounds relatively slowly. Those who reduce slowly tend to lose more fat and less muscle.[16]

- People are about ten times more likely to change on their own than to be helped by doctors, therapists, or self-help groups. Spontaneity works better than highly structured plans. Inner changes are more important to long-term weight balance than diet and exercise changes.[15]

- An eight-year experience with a very-low-calorie diet formula for the control of major obesity, with multidisciplinary group counseling, found that 25 percent of the patients were unable to adapt to this approach, dropping out within the first three weeks, with only 5 to 10 percent maintaining weight loss after 18 months.[17]

- Those who go on so-called "starvation" or restricted calorie diets end up spending a great amount of time thinking about food and weight, which in turn is related to weight increases, not weight loss.[18] In addition, there is evidence that a restricted weight loss diet may lead to mental and emotional personality disturbances similar to those exhibited in people who are starving, and causing people to perform cruel, malicious and mean acts. In such cases, depression, irritability, anxiety, pessimism and anger frequently persist during recovery for six months or even more.[19]

- As reported in *American Health Magazine*, Market Data Enterprises, a market research company, compiled data on thousands of patients in several of the major liquid diet programs. A year or more after completing a program, up to 60 percent had regained their weight. Add the large number who never finished the programs, and it is clear that chances for sustained weight loss are slim.

- Patients will regain significant amounts of weight, even with multidisciplinary care.[20]

- A study of relapse crises and coping among dieters showed that dieters who were emotionally upset almost always resorted back to overeating.[21]

- Of 400 patients in maintenance following treatment with supplemented fasting and behavior modification for three months, 55 percent discontinued prior to completing the program. Those who completed the treatment lost 84 percent of their initial excess weight, but regained 59 to 82 percent of their initial excess weight within 30 months.[22]

- People have lost weight using purely behavioral approaches, but rarely as much as 40 pounds. And just like people who lose weight with liquid diets, jaw-wiring, or other techniques, they tend to gain it back. With very low calorie diets and intense behavior therapy, things really fall apart by three years, with only a small number of participants not regaining all but ten pounds of the weight they've lost.[23]

- A San Diego State University analysis of a very low-calorie diet plus behavior modification revealed that less than half of a group of 400 dieters completed the program. Those who did complete it regained 70 to 100 percent of the lost weight within 30 months.[24]

- Dr. Ralph D'Agostino of Boston University and the famous Framingham Heart Study, reported that in a 32-year collection of data of 3000 subjects who were 10 pounds overweight, there was found to be a 50 percent greater risk of heart disease.[25] In addition, when a person's weight fluctuates by 10 or more pounds, such as is common with yo-yo dieting through weight loss programs, he or she is at a 200 percent greater risk of developing heart disease.

- In October 1990, Dr. Philip A. Kern and others of the Cedars-Sinai Medical Center in Los Angeles stated his research indicated that obese people have overactive lipoprotein lipase (LPL), a special enzyme that metabolizes fat (i.e., which stuffs fat), and that rapid weight loss doubled LPL activity, meaning a certain regain of lost weight after very-low calorie-diets.[26]

CONGRESS CHECKS TRUTH AND SAFETY

These readings are but a small sample of results from the research literature available today. Some additional and trustworthy findings have become available to the public as a result of several congressional investigations. Although the investigations don't restrict the weight loss industry, they do suggest guidelines for truth in advertising regarding long-term success of their products and services. The fraud and lack of efficacy prevalent in the weight loss industry are clear.

Hearings were held in the spring of 1990 under the chairmanship of Representative Ron Wyden from Oregon, and under the auspices of a group known as the House Subcommittee on Regulation, Business Opportunities, and Energy Dealing with Health, Safety and Consumer Protection Issues Involving Weightloss Programs. These hearings and the FTC hearings of 1998 show us the physical damage, economic loss, and extremely poor effectiveness of weight loss efforts in the long-term. They also demonstrate how the individual consumer's self-efficacy is undermined by dependence on these inadequate programs. Following are a few important excerpts from the congressional findings.

- The American Medical Association's Council on Scientific Affairs warned, "the zealous marketing of various formula products to physicians, as well as the public's appetite for such diets, could lead to yet another round of complications and fatalities." (See Dr. Callaway's testimony presented later in this section.)

  - Most experts agree that fast weight loss is dangerous in and of itself. Very low calorie liquid diets are the principal concern of the council—and also one of the fastest growing segments of the weight loss industry.

  - Research now suggests that starving inevitably leads to stuffing. The weight is gained back faster, and it is lost more slowly the next time around.

- Sixty percent of medical school graduates don't get adequate training in nutrition, often leaving them without even a basic understanding of the complicated physiological and psychological factors in obesity, according to the Association of American Medical Colleges. Related facts arising from the hearings include:

  - It is a public misconception that the experts know what they are doing. Despite their medical degrees, most physicians know little about how to treat the overweight and obese.

  - Liquid diet manufactures aggressively market their wares to doctors. A sample come-on suggests that a physician can net over $22,000 yearly treating only 20 patients, and over $70,000 by treating 100.

  - NutriSystems CEO A. Donald McCulloch admitted that his nutrition specialists and behavior counselors get just one week of company training.

  - Dr. Jerry Sutkamp, Medical Director of Physicians Weightloss Centers, stated: "Our physicians have no special training in nutrition other then what they receive in medical school."

- According to the Surgeon General's Report on Health and Nutrition, the causes of obesity are poorly understood and, therefore, knowledge about how to prevent and treat it is also limited.

  - Medical management of obesity is almost universally unsuccessful.

  - Another public misconception is that if these programs were dangerous, the government would stop it.

The Food and Drug Administration (FDA) is sitting on the side lines. Nearly 30 years ago, the FDA began drafting regulations on over-the-counter weight loss products. The resulting monograph was finally published in 1982. Eighteen years later, that monograph still rests, unimplemented, in the bowels of the FDA's bureaucracy.

THE SLEEPING WATCHDOG

State medical boards testifying before the FTC subcommittee nine years ago said that their state attorneys general told them not to police weight loss ads because they would be sued by the FTC for restraint-of-trade. While the FTC has focused on print advertising, it has left radio and television advertising—which most of the biggest plans use to sell their products— totally alone.

In February of 1999, the FTC set up The Partnership for Healthy Weight Management. This partnership is a coalition composed of representatives from science, academia, the health care professions, government, commercial enterprises, and organizations promoting the public interest. Out of this gathering has come the *Voluntary Guidelines for Providers of Weight Loss Products or Services*, which was referred to earlier.

C. Wayne Callaway, M.D., from George Washington University and the American Board of Nutrition, testified before the FTC on March 26, 1990. Some of the impressive comments from his testimony follow:

- "Commercial weightloss programs do not exist in a vacuum. They are skillfully and deliberately exploiting a situation where cultural norms are dramatically out of sync with biological reality. Sudden deaths still occur. The fact that we have not heard about them until recently reflects our lack of any type of tracking mechanism. We have no way of knowing how common these occurrences are. When the victim or her survivors have raised legal issues, the cases have generally been settled out of court and the documents sealed. It is only when the media attention is brought to bear on this problem, as occurred with the extremely high frequency of gallstones in people on low-calorie diets, that victims recognize that they are not simply isolated cases. The *Archives of Internal Medicine* show that in eight weeks of dieting on a 500 calorie diet, 25 percent of dieters developed gallstones."

- Symptoms of high protein liquid fast diets include fatigue, depression, sleep abnormalities, cold intolerance, dry skin, dry hair, loss of hair, constipation, delayed emptying of solid food from the stomach, a fall in blood pressure associated with dizziness and even loss of consciousness on standing, and alterations in perceptions of time and space. Dieting leads to binge eating, with no mention in the commercial promotions that fatal irregularities in heartbeat could result from prolonged semi-starvation.

- Hospital-based programs which hire part-time, untrained physicians should also bear responsibility for the adverse outcomes.

In addition to the statements from the investigating team, government agencies, commercial weight loss program representatives, and those of us who had worked with or for these programs, there were also testimonies from consumers of these products and programs. Two of these individuals served to illustrate some of the dangers of quick weight loss.

- One was the mother of a Loretta, a 13-year-old girl. Loretta was put on a very-low-calorie diet at a "doctor supervised" center for quick weight loss. This diet resulted in an emergency operation to remove Loretta's gallbladder.

- The second was the wife of a 44-year-old Ph.D., a university professor of engineering. The woman described how her husband had utilized a quick weight loss packaged food program and followed the diet to the letter, exercising faithfully. He had a near fatal heart attack and ended up in a coma which resulted in permanent damage to both his short- and long-term memory. He will never be able to work or live independently again. He has lost all of his technical knowledge and his daily activities now must be planned for him. His emotional affect has been significantly impaired to the point that he cannot respond to his family in a sensitive, loving way. He lost all this and his income for life—a very big price for 30 pounds of unwanted weight.

REFERENCES

1. Koop CE: "U.S. Surgeon General's Report on Nutrition and Health, 1988." Available from the Office of Disease Prevention and Health Promotion, Communication Support Center, P.O. Box 37366, Washington DC 20013-8366; telephone (301) 468-5960.

2. Wolf AM and GA Colditz: "Current Estimates of the Economic Cost of Obesity in the United States." *Obesity Research*, Mar 1998; 6(2): 97-106.

3. Satcher D: letter to the author, 1998.

4. Friedman JM: "Obesity in the New Millennium." *Nature*, Apr 6, 2000; 404(6778): 632-634.

5. Federal Trade Commission: "Voluntary Guidelines for Providers of Weight Loss Products or Services," February, 1999. Available online at: *http://www.ftc.gov/bcp/conline/pubs/buspubs/wgtguide.htm*, 9/22/00.

6. Federal Trade Commission: "Commercial Weight Loss Products and Programs What Consumers Stand To Gain and Lose." Report on Conference, Washington, DC; Oct 16-17, 1997. Available online at: *http://www.ftc.gov/os/1998/9803/weightlo.rpt.htm*, 9/25/00.

7. Davidson MH, et al.: "Weight Control and Risk Factor Reduction in Obese Subjects Treated for 2 Years with Orlistat: a Randomized Controlled Trial." *JAMA*, Apr 7, 1999; 281(13) 1174.

8. Physicians Committee for Responsible Medicine: *Good Medicine*, Spring 1999, 8(2).

9. "Manufacturer Settles Suit in Fen-Phen User's Death." *Arizona Republic*, Jun 23, 1999, p. A5.

10. "Weight-Loss Pill Firm Must Repay $8 Million." *Arizona Republic*, Jul 20, 1999.

11. Fatis M, et al.: "Following Up on a Commercial Weight Loss Program: Do the Pounds Stay Off after Your Picture Has Been in the Newspaper?" *Journal of the American Dietetic Association*, Apr 1989; 89(4): 547-548.

12. *Nation's Business*, July 1989.

13. Bray GA and DS Gray: "Obesity Part II: Treatment." *Western Journal of Medicine*, Nov 1988; 149(5): 555-571.

14. Wadden TA, et al.: "Treatment of Obesity by Very Low Calorie Diet, Behavior Therapy, and Their Combination: A Five-Year Perspective." *International Journal of Obesity*, 1989; 13(Suppl 2): 39-46.

15. Forest J: "Fighting Fat: A Three-Day Report." *USA Today*, February 1990.

16. Korkeila M, et al.: "Weight-loss Attempts and Risk of Major Weight Gain: A Prospective Study in Finnish Adults." *American Journal of Clinical Nutrition*, Dec 1999; 70(6): 965-975.

17. Kirschner MA, et al.: "An Eight-Year Experience with a Very-Low-Calorie Formula Diet for Control of Major Obesity." *International Journal of Obesity*, 1988; 12(1):69-80.

18. Berg F: "Thinking Too Much about Food." *Healthy Weight Journal*, Nov/Dec 1998; 12(6). Available online at: *http://www.healthyweightnetwork.com/editor.htm*, 9/22/00.

19. Berg F: "Living in Starvation Mode." *Healthy Weight Journal*, Sep/Oct 1998; 12(5). Available online at: *http://www.healthyweightnetwork.com/editor.htm*, 9/22/00.

20. Kopelman PG: "Obesity as a Medical Problem." *Nature*, Apr 6, 2000; 404(6778): 634-643.

21. Bliss RE, et al.: "Relapse Crises and Coping among Dieters." *Journal of Counseling and Clinical Psychology*, Aug 1989; 57(4): 488-495.

22. Hovell MF, et al.: "Long-Term Weight Loss Maintenance: Assessment of a Behavioral and Supplemented Fasting Regimen." *American Journal of Public Health*, Jun 1988; 78(6): 663-666.

23. *Psychology Today*, June 1989.

24. *American Health Magazine*, March 1989.

25. Lissner L, et al.: "Variability of Body Weight and Health Outcomes in the Framingham Population." *New England Journal of Medicine*, Jun 27, 1991; 324(26): 1839-1844.

26. Kern PA: "The Effects of Weight Loss on the Activity and Expression of Adipose-Tissue Lipoprotein Lipase in Very Obese Humans." *New England Journal of Medicine*, Apr 12, 1990; 322(15): 1053-1059.

Chapter 1

HOW DID I GET HERE?

Figuring Out How It Happened Is
Knowing What to Change

*L*ouise watched from outside the screen door, fearful that her drunk father would hit her mother again. She was torn with emotions. She felt overwhelmed by guilt; feeling that somehow this was all her fault, and that she should be helping her mother. But she was afraid that her dad would leave for good if she tried to help her mother, and that both of them would leave her if she couldn't make things better at home.

She was the baby. Always in the way. The one her older sister blamed for having to stay home to cook and clean instead of having fun with her friends. Louise's mother worked long and hard to support the family, but was always mad and yelling at her dad. Louise's father responded by getting drunk, gambling, running around with other women, and beating his wife. Louise was sure it was all her fault and wouldn't have blamed her sister or parents if they wanted to leave her. The only thing she felt she could do was to be as good and as helpful and as non-demanding as possible, with the hope that then her family wouldn't want to leave her.

Louise promised herself that she would never show anger like her dad and that she would always work hard like her mother. She could make people laugh. She knew what pleased her father when he was angry. She knew that she could keep her sister happy—and even get to go places with her occasionally—if she asked for nothing and did some of her sister's chores. Her mother was critical and demanding and left Louise feeling that she could never quite please her, no matter how hard she tried.

Both of Louise's parents were perfectionists, manifesting feelings of shame and guilt by being critical and demanding of their children, particularly Louise—who, with her lack of self-esteem and feelings of guilt, was a vulnerable target.

For a long time, a fear had been deeply instilled in Louise. This fear kept her anxious and on guard for more than twenty years: it was the on-going fear that she would never be quite good enough and that she must always put others above herself; the belief that she must learn what pleased others, and the feeling of guilt if she couldn't please them. Louise's entire life experience had left her ill-prepared to get to know or nurture herself or to believe in her worth.

While Louise was growing up, all the people she depended on the most modeled the behavior that crushed her belief in herself and taught her how to be the consummate people-pleaser who stuffed her anger with the only thing that comforted her: a "hug from the refrigerator." With the refrigerator supplying all of her hugs, Louise was about twenty pounds overweight by the time she was twelve. She was shy and quiet but, of course, well-liked, because she was funny, selfless, and appeared to be happy.

Different, Yet the Same

Other heavy people may grow up in very different circumstances from those of Louise, with parents who are educated, who don't drink or gamble, who do not physically or emotionally abuse them, and who are supportive of their activities, but who show subtle, underlying expectations that achieving or winning is what approval is all about. To young children, it appears as though their performance defines their worth.

The psychodynamics of how you might have developed into a person who is apt to be compulsive, overweight, and suffering from low self-esteem and on-going anxiety and perfectionism to the point of diminishing returns, can easily be seen by going over the following six steps and analyzing what in your developmental years may have led to what seems to be an uncontrollable, chronic weight problem.

1. Root causes

2. Thought patterns

3. Dominant resulting emotions

4. Self-concept development

5. Basic motivations

6. Behavior patterns

As you study each of the six steps, reflect on your years from childhood to the present. Then ask yourself and/or other family members who know you well if any of these conditions existed to the extent that they would lead to the behaviors described in Step 6. Check off those items which seem to apply to your own life.

The Psycho/Sociodynamics of the Emotional and Behavioral Development of the Overweight Personality

1. Root Causes:

   _ Genetic predisposition, culture, and family customs

   _ Limited or qualified praise from parents and significant others

   _ High expectations of your parents for you or others

   _ Perfectionist parents

   _ Overprotective or dominating parent or parents

   _ First born in your family

   _ A role model of an older sibling(s) who is a high achiever

   _ Verbal, physical, or sexual abuse by adults

   _ Family handicaps: social, emotional, physical, financial, educational

   _ Environmental conditioning pertaining to eating habits and a negative self-concept

   _ Shortage of information about healthful eating and exercise

The presence of one or more of the above conditions in your formative years may lead to one or more of the following:

2. Thought patterns:

   _ Disordered thinking (busy mind; hard to complete a thought)

   _ Poor self-awareness

   _ Narrow perspective (limited or incomplete view of life and the world)

   _ Critical or negative thinking

   _ Close-minded, or frightened or angered by new ideas

   _ Defensive; avoid challenges

   _ High expectations of self and others

   _ Parent message (shoulds, musts, have-to-be's)

   _ Over-simplifying or catastrophizing (i.e., all or nothing)

   _ Indecision (insecure conflict about what "is right")

   _ External focus (give more attention to others than to self)

   _ Denial or suppression of life's realities

   _ Achievement-oriented (if you achieve enough, problems will dissolve)

One or more of these thought patterns will usually lead to one or more of the following:

3. Dominant resulting emotions:

   _ Fear of failure, rejection, being unloved

   _ Guilt about what you do or don't do

   _ Anxiety or impatience, often without awareness or acknowledgement

   _ Frustration and contained anger

   _ Hurt and disappointment; hypersensitivity

   _ Loneliness and depression; low energy

_ Manic (exaggerated, short-term happiness)

One or more of these dominant emotions will usually lead to one or more of the following:

4. Self-concept development:

    _ Low self-worth, self-esteem, and/or self-trust

    _ Feelings of inadequacy and dependence

    _ Feelings of helplessness and/or hopelessness

    _ Feel valued only as an achiever

One or more of these self-image beliefs will usually lead to a reliance on one or more of the following:

5. Basic motivations:

    _ Affiliation (closely associated in a dependent or subordinate way)

    _ Achievement (to acquire affiliation)

    _ Power (to control people and circumstances to be perfect)

Finally, one or more factors in each of the previous five steps may have contributed to one or more of the following behavior patterns:

6. Behavior patterns:

    _ Compulsive, need structure, focus on detail, narrow focus

    _ Procrastinate and/or avoid

    _ Perfectionist in thinking and behavior

    _ Strive to please those those outside the family (i.e., people-pleasing behavior)

    _ Critical, nagging, and accusing with self and family

    _ Controlling, pushy, manipulative

    _ Hyperactive or sedentary

    _ Have difficulty accepting new ideas

    _ Have difficulty letting go of people, ideas, possessions

    _ Easily conditioned by external events and circumstances

_ Neglectful of self to win approval of others.

As important as the family is in the development of a chronic weight problem, other heavily influencing factors must also be considered. The family unit is, after all, part of a much larger community, regional, country, and now global environment that constantly lets us know what is expected of us, what we must be and do to be accepted, approved of, and rewarded—in short, all the things most people want and are willing to work and perform for; standards we are told to achieve and live by.

If you haven't noticed, we live in a very fast-paced, competitive world that is becoming more so each day. Dealing with personal achievements, traffic, job, school, social activities and keeping up with the world and what goes on around us is demanding. It almost assures that we will be spending a great percentage of our time focusing on externals so as not to be swept away in the current of life; that we will have little time to know or understand ourselves; and finally, that we must be on guard most of the time so we will lose as few rounds as possible. Especially for the overweight person with low self-esteem, losing is the ultimate fear. To lose social acceptance is to face rejection or the withholding of a reward.

With the prospects of being swept away, with fear of loss and rejection always hanging over everyone's heads, the person who has been taught at home not to trust, believe in, or like himself or herself is going to be much more anxious and will try much harder to be perfect or to avoid as many challenges as possible. Under these everyday conditions, stress becomes an ongoing way of life; yet we may not be aware of it and therefore don't do anything about it. Subconsciously, then, we turn to food. Because it is sensually comforting, and because taste and aroma create neurochemical reactions in the brain that lead to pleasurable feelings, food can easily become the drug of choice to calm oneself. Of course, when stress is ongoing, a great deal of sensual comfort is necessary—and many hugs from the refrigerator are sought.

Many of us grew up with a shortage of information about food and exercise, and even now we are only starting to understand the effects of food on our physical and emotional well-being. To stay abreast of the new research and follow all the debates on how to interpret the findings is intimidating—it feels like one needs a Ph.D., not to mention an enormous amount of free time, in order to analyze and understand the information. But, in fact, such a commitment is unnecessary. The individuals who have lost weight and kept it off over the long term and through their own efforts found the information they needed very easy to access (see Chapter 9, "The 5-Plus Club").

Our culture continues to give us many destructive messages about food; e.g., steak and apple pie are "the American way." Not only are many of our conditioning messages destructive, they are also conflicting. The media bombards us with the message that trim is in, while at the same time they promote all kinds of appealing, high-calorie, non-nutritious food. We're also encouraged to strive to be the best, the richest, the most beautiful, and the happiest. But the truth is, if you achieve those goals but are unable to remain stress-free, you won't even be able to enjoy your successes. The twisted messages continue, implying that if you do manage to out-perform many people, you should feel guilty and must push yourself even harder to give a great deal back to those who you've worked so hard to outpace.

With all the straining, conflict, confusion, guilt, and shame about what we aren't and what should be driving us to be compulsive, we long for sensual comfort and reach for food. Resisting it is more than having the proper information and overcoming genetic predisposition and cultural conditioning. It's more than simply eating fewer calories and expending more energy.

Louise, for example, was taught from childhood to be a perfectionist. Although in recent years she has became aware of the relationship between straining to be perfect and her weight problem, she was still faced with doing many things to bring about self-change. For starters, se had to determine what type of perfectionist she was, to what extent her perfectionism related to her weight problem, and how to go about modifying her perfectionist traits.

Louise's understanding of how she came to be the person she is has been extremely helpful in her understanding of why she made the choices about her life and lifestyle that kept her overweight for so long. She is now more aware and sensitive to what she is doing and feeling at the time she is doing it. If nothing else, this awareness gives her the choice to change old behaviors that didn't work for her. As time has gone on, her awareness has increased and Louise has become more willing to risk change. She is still a perfectionist, but much less so than she was. Her perfectionism is not as self-defeating, and as she becomes increasingly satisfied with her efforts to change she will be less fearful of making the next changes.

Chapter 2

THE FAT PERSONALITY

Who We Are Might
Tip the Scales

*R*are *are the days that Louise does not appear at work without her* beautiful smile, flawless skin, rosy cheeks, and quick, self-effacing sense of humor. She is always interested in the well-being of her close friends and colleagues; and she is a hard worker, eager to do more than her share without a complaint and with seldom an error. She is modest, sensitive to the feelings of others, and generous to a fault.

It is hard to guess that she is in pain most of the time with a serious back injury, frequent migraine headaches, and a lump in her breast that the doctors monitor closely. Nor would you know that she has a family of four adults at home that count on her to keep everything in their lives together. In return, they provide her with so little intimacy that loneliness is her closest friend. Yet, her complaints are few.

Louise's co-worker, Tomi, is also highly respected at work. Her performance, too, is without fault. However, she is quick to criticize, although usually not aloud. Her smiles are few and her stoic responses to humor stop most jokes cold. Unlike Louise, she has developed few close friends and does not appear sensitive to the pain of others. Also unlike Louise, she is aggressive and very competitive. At home, she kicks the dog and yells at her kids and her husband, who can never seem to please her. She controls with an iron hand and complains endlessly about the problems of her life, namely: work, home, husband, and kids.

Both Louise and Tomi are small in stature and between 40 and 50 pounds overweight. What might surprise you is that they also have a strong commonality in their personalities. Both Louise and Tomi, like 85 percent or more of the clients I have seen for chronic weight problems, are perfectionists. Louise and Tomi represent different manifestations of the same personality type: the perfectionist.

Like most perfectionists, their focus is outward, watching the world and all in it to gauge what is expected of them. They are always on guard and ready, so as not to fail. Falling short of expectations in any way means more than disappointment for them. It also means embarrassment, anger, guilt, shame, rejection, or the ultimate failure of not being loved.

Approval is everything to perfectionists! Most of their motivation and satisfaction come from outside themselves in the form of approval or perceived rejection. This leads to the belief that *in performance is their only worth*. Once this idea is established, it is only a question of how to perform to win others' approval.

Each perfectionist may approach this in a somewhat different way, as you can see by looking at Louise and Tomi. Louise is the avoider. She avoids conflict and challenge and pushes her real feelings much deeper than Tomi. She blames herself more, has more feelings of guilt, and admits to feelings of inadequacy more easily. She presents herself as more passive and willing to defer and she seeks ways to please people as much as possible. Louise feels much more secure and happy when she receives reinforcement that her ways have won acceptance.

Tomi, on the other hand, is aggressive and tries to control rather than defer to others. She focuses more on the rules to prove she can't be blamed or officially rejected. Tomi would resist admitting any feelings of inadequacy, and rather than trying to win social approval, she is more apt to use intimidation. She finds it easier to blame others and to rationalize her position. Like Louise, she avoids those things she is sure she can't do well. Unlike Louise, she "puts down" those things and the people who do them. Louise admires and praises those who do what she thinks she would find too difficult.

Overweight perfectionists, like all perfectionists, are prone to have more difficulty with their emotions, as they have high expectations for themselves, and high expectations of others as well. In Tomi's case, this is especially true of her expectations of her children and husband. Perfectionists' expectations set them up to be more vulnerable to negative emotions and resistant to change. Tomi looks for things to go wrong and attempts to avoid error by straining to be perfect, which she is sure won't be good enough. While procrastination is more common among avoiders like Louise, it tends to be true of aggressive types like Tomi, too. Putting things off until the last minute gives one less time to prepare. Then, if things don't turn out well, a weak performance can be considered acceptable due to the lack of adequate preparation time. It won't be considered a failure. If the performance comes out well in spite of minimal preparation, the procrastinator is fantastic. Either way, the perfectionist/procrastinator is safe. There is no risk of failure.

One question these ideas may invite is: if overweight perfectionists are always focused on meeting the perceived expectations of others, why would the obese person allow himself or herself to take the chance of rejection by remaining obese?

Because they have learned to work extra hard to please people or to be "right," they are unlikely to be rejected. And, if rejection does come, they can blame their obesity. Because we know the stigma attached to obesity almost assures weak or low self esteem, which in turn contributes to low self-worth, it is easy to see why a person like Louise is more apt to feel guilty giving herself the same time and attention she always gives to others. Her own physical needs are therefore postponed. We all need approval and praise from others, as well as ourselves, and if we only get this approval for what we do for others, we may let our own needs slide. In addition, someone like Tomi may believe that if she does achieve a trim body, she'll face new, uncontrollable challenges she could not handle. By holding on to her fat, she avoids facing these challenges.

Perfectionists like Louise and Tomi are more subject to stress and distress, which leads to what Dom Deluise's cookbook states so profoundly, "Eat This. You'll Feel Better!"

THE FAT PERSONALITY QUIZ

Please answer "yes" or "no" to the following questions:

1. Do you routinely set aside your own personal needs to be the best at school or work or to please other people? _____

2. Do people who know you very well describe you as a perfectionist? _____

3. When people around you are upset, bored, or in difficulty, do you feel a responsibility to fix things for them? _____

4. Do you frequently contain your feelings to avoid criticism, except at home? _____

5. Are you quick to criticize yourself or others, or both? _____

6. Do you usually push to be the best at what you do, or avoid doing anything at which you may not excel? _____

7. When you have a fear that limits the quality of your life, do you seldom initiate moving toward the fear to get it resolved? _____

8. Do you strain, quit, or become very tense when you know you are being compared with others? _____

9. Do you often feel depressed about your weight? _____

10. Do you become anxious or bored, especially when you are not "productive"? _____

11. Is most change in your life difficult for you? _____

12. If you lose excess weight, do you wonder if you'll keep it off?

    _____

13. Do you want a high degree of structure and time to prepare before you can feel comfortable in new situations? _____

14. Are you easily hurt, angered, or made to feel guilty? _____

15. Do you push for control, fear being controlled, fear loss of control, or think you want to be controlled? (If any are true, answer "yes".) _____

16. Have you known yourself to rebel, openly or otherwise, when you knew it was in your best interest not to? _____

17. Is anger or touching hard for you to deal with? _____

18. Do you often respond to your emotions by eating? _____

19. Do you use food to express love, reward, or to punish yourself? _____

20. Do you eat more or differently when you are alone? _____

21. Do you plan to keep your food taste preferences as they are? _____

22. Do you benefit—have advantages or security—by being over-weight? _____

23. Do you have less than one enjoyable sexual release each week? _____

24. Do you believe you'll need help to lose your extra weight and keep it off? _____

25. Is losing weight more important and urgent to you than changing self-defeating personality traits? _____

Total the number of "yes" answers. The numbers will indicate the following:

0-7   *You are likely to stay trim or lose weight easily*

8-16   *Weight gain may be easy and weight loss very hard to maintain*

17-25   *Personality trait changes must precede any long-term success in keeping weight in balance with height and build*

The perfectionist personality is not the only aspect of the fat personality, it is simply the most common characteristic in the chronically overweight people with whom I have worked over the years. All of the questions in the "Fat Personality Quiz" are also aspects that can be found in a variety of other personality groupings, such as the compulsive/addictive types, which also fits with the co-dependent/caretaker, anxiety/depressive types, and certainly, anorexic/bulimic types. None of these classifications, or any other, will fit any one person exactly, or should I say, "perfectly." Each individual is still unique, just as are Louise and Tomi. It is only theoretically and statistically useful to bring commonalities together under a single label for the sake of clarifying the overall larger problem.

The larger problem is that more than 95 percent of the people who utilize external assistance to lose weight—such as surgical techniques, fasting programs, packaged foods, behavioral groups, hormone shots, diets, pills, health food store supplements, hypnosis, gimmicks and equipment of every kind—regain their weight plus more within five years (usually much sooner), if they stay with any program long enough to lose a significant amount of weight to begin with. Personality has a great deal to do with why the overweight person procrastinates, has difficulty staying motivated, drops out, or sabotages his or her own efforts. Personality, values, conditioning, attitudes, beliefs, preferences, habits, emotional needs, motivations and choices are interrelated.

Chapter 3

SELF-SABOTAGING

"Why Don't I Do What
I Think I Want to Do, When
I Know How to Do It?"

*L**ouise did, and does, know the basics of how to lose weight. Her* education in nutrition and exercise, as well as about a wide variety of weight-loss techniques, was certainly more than adequate. Louise had been aware of the psycho-social dynamics described in Chapter 1, and the "fat personality" traits described in Chapter 2 for a long time. If Louise hadn't changed, it certainly wasn't because she lacked information.

With each new weight loss program, method, or technique, Louise planned and organized. She would buy the products and supplies necessary to achieve her goals (i.e., tread mill, books, proper food). She would go to class, and set up times and places to pull it all together. She then would usually make a consistent effort for a week or two. Her initial enthusiasm would be high and would fade only gradually, usually even after all her efforts had come to an end. In fact, I finally noticed in conversations much later that she would still unnecessarily defend the method and her plan and blame herself for failing. Louise, as it turns out, did the same things with weight-loss methods, products, diets, or gurus as she did with her father, mother, and sister. When things went wrong, she felt guilty, inadequate, and to blame. Even in our private counseling sessions she would apologize for everything from speaking first or holding a different opinion to taking more than a few brief minutes to explain her thoughts. If I just looked at her for a few moments without expression or comment, she would blush, smile her defensive, "I'm sorry" smile, become very nervous and stumble over her words, acting like a child caught with her hand in the cookie jar, and apologizing in a voice that was both short of breath (tightened throat) and so soft it was almost inaudible.

Louise's fear of rejection was plain to almost anyone and more extreme than in most people I see, but what wasn't so clear was the anger that the constricted throat was holding back. The blush, the smile, the apology, and the cute little-girl way of phrasing things all covered up the anger, so most people would not notice. Many other people with fat personalities display their anger, and the fear behind it is overlooked, but Louise was the avoider. From early childhood, Louise had been stuffing and eating her anger, until it was hard for her to even imagine allowing herself to acknowledge anger, let alone express it fully and openly.

Every day, millions of people do what Louise did, maybe not in the same manner, degree, or time. They avoid being in touch with their feelings and deny their anger, expressing it only after it has built up to an explosion. Then they may direct their anger mostly at people they think they love and are dependent on, usually family members and pets.

Playing the role of people-pleaser, caretaker, or co-dependent and deferring one's personal needs for days, weeks, months, or even years results in a buildup of anger, resentment and frustration. Always putting personal needs aside to pacify or please others leaves one feeling cheated, lonely, unloved or uncared for. Emotional pressure will build and find some way out, if not in an uncontrolled explosion, certainly in other ways.

The intellectual mind says, "I've learned not to make others angry," so you rationalize not expressing yourself. Since you can't be blamed for what you can't control, you express your anger in a passive-aggressive manner way by rebelling and not losing weight. You're innocent. You didn't get mad at "them" directly. You just got back at them by not losing the weight "they" wanted you to lose.

No, this doesn't make sense, but emotions don't have to make sense. The behavior and the emotions that go with the behavior keep the mind games going and, even more, they keep the overweight person from dealing with challenges, questions, and problems that are frightening to them.

Louise's situation illustrates only one of endless ways people can play games with their weight. Power, fear, denial, rebellion, control, vengeance, and reward are a few more behaviors and mind games emotional people get into about their weight. None of them needs to have a great deal of logic or reason. But after all, the perfectionists live most their lives trying to do the "right" thing. Food sometimes seems like the only comfort or sanctuary the perfectionist has. Then too, the perfectionists are much more prone to be emotionally stressed, and emotions are a more powerful motivator than logic. A bright mind can justify self-sabotaging behaviors and staying overweight as being the right thing to do.

Each person has his or her own special reasons and set of circumstances for what he or she is doing or not doing, and if change is to come about, these reasons need to be clarified, accepted, and dealt with by their owner. From a base of low self-esteem, it is hard enough just to examine the difficult questions, let alone acknowledge the blocks, identify the means of getting past them and, in a gradual, self-initiated way, take the action needed to bring about lasting changes.

Let's talk about a few people other than Louise, and look at why, with all the personal differences, one commonality always exists which seems to be the major stumbling block or the point at which taking action to change stops.

Mr. B. puffed with pride as he told me he earned $250,000 a year as an attorney and had a beautiful home and an intelligent, attractive wife. He belonged to all the right clubs, bought a new, expensive car every two years, traveled all over the world, and had sent his two kids to the best colleges. He was also very proud that he had graduated near the top of his class at Yale. Undoubtedly, this was a very bright man.

When he came into my office, Mr. B. was somewhat defensive, feeling demeaned for being there, and attempting to minimize his need for assistance. If sixty extra pounds weren't so hard to conceal, I'm sure he would not have been in my office at all! However, his weight wasn't his only problem. His doctor had also told him that he had hypertension, ulcers, colitis and, at age 45, he wasn't likely to see 50 if he didn't deal with his weight, drinking and job stress. Although Mr. B. told me that his clients, colleagues, and friends at the club loved him, thought he was funny and a master at his profession, his wife was on the verge of filing for divorce, and his kids only talked to him when they needed money.

Yes, Mr. B. was a people-pleaser. He was focused completely outwardly, always ready to jump to meet the next expectation, and he was highly anxious, depressed and confused as to why his life was a nightmare. He could not understand why he was so unhappy, and why, when he was so successful in most areas of his life, his family life was so miserable. Unlike Louise, he had a litany of blame for other people and for situations he couldn't "control."

He was going to give me a chance, he warned, but I had better be practical, organized, businesslike and quick, or he wouldn't be around long. To win his confidence and encourage his continuing efforts, I suggested that he respond to his wife's next daily threat to leave not by defending himself, but by acknowledging and showing understanding for her complaints and threats to leave. I knew this sudden change would shock and confuse her, and she would back off, at least for awhile—which she did—and I gained the time and confidence I needed from him.

Mr. B. took notes and followed all the practical weight-loss suggestions I made, and, of course, for that period when he was taking those steps, he lost the desired weight. Knowing this small improvement would only be temporary, I gradually started to probe into more sensitive and important matters. As I did so, his defenses would rise accordingly until finally he would accept the new ideas and again calm down.

Mr.B. could acknowledge that he was a perfectionist, and a "damn good one." He was proud of it. He had achieved all his success by being a perfectionist. It was why his reputation at work and the club was so good. He owed everything to his perfectionism. It was very hard for him to see the huge price he was paying and had always paid for his perfectionism. It took him a long time to admit his perfectionism was resulting in:

- *Decreased productivity and inability to reach desired goals.*
  Like many athletes, he did very well, but always fell short of his capabilities. He was slowed down by attempting precision, being redundant, and missing the big picture.

- *Impaired health.* Straining to be the best and fearing he wouldn't be, Mr. B. was always anxious, in addition to not having time to take care of himself because it would take time away from his performance for others. The constant strain weakened his immune system and overtaxed his whole body. Distress and health don't mix.

- *Serious mood disorders,* such as high anxiety and depression. Loneliness, obsessive compulsiveness, disordered thinking, and even suicidal thoughts may occur in this circle of self-defeating thinking and behavior.

- *Poor self-control.* Distress means heightened emotions—the higher the emotions, the less the control. The more unreasonable the expectations and the lower the self-esteem, the more he saw his difficulties as hopeless.

- *Troubled relationships.* It is not easy to like someone who is often critical, puts himself down, becomes depressed and anxious easily, and expects others us to be as perfect as he thinks he "should" be.

- *Low self-esteem.* Low self-esteem meant that Mr. B. believed his only worth was his performance. In other words, if his performance was not perfect, he was a failure. Straining to be perfect, he continually fell short of the goal (at least in his perception). Then he would put himself down, and the cycle would repeat.

- *Procrastination.* Because he believed he was likely to fail in an attempt to lose weight (fall short of perfect), he was avoiding or postponing doing any thing about it.

Accepting the price he paid for his perfectionism didn't necessarily mean Mr. B. was ready to work on modifying his perfectionist traits. Mr. B. believed that his perfectionist behavior and thinking were responsible for his success in life, and to change his approach could mean he would lose everything, including his wife and kids. It was very hard for him to believe that if he were more centered and balanced, maintained an intrinsic as opposed to an extrinsic focus, lowered his expectations, and was less critical of himself, then he would do even better with work, friends, clients, and money. As it was, his perfectionism meant he was so focused on others that he had lost a great deal of self-awareness.

He could understand it intellectually but could not internalize it on an emotional level. The only way Mr. B. ever would be able to internalize it would be if he experienced himself doing things differently. Faced with the fear of changing, Mr. B., like so many others, stopped his efforts and slowly slipped back to his old weight. Unfortunately, it is unlikely that he ever will be able to make the shifts necessary to sustain true change.

Real change means facing the unknown on one's own terms over a long and gradual time period. We believe about ourselves what we see ourselves do. Repeatedly experiencing new behavior which is self-directed allows us to eventually internalize what is intellectually understood. The person has changed.

People have different fears to face. For example, some women believe that if they become thinner and more physically attractive they will have men pursuing them. They fear that they might succumb to promiscuity, risking their marriages. In truth, they would be less apt to become promiscuous, because they would no longer have to be people-pleasers. They would balance their logic and emotions and make better decisions. Their self-esteem would be enhanced, and they would no longer see their performance as their only worth. Expectations of others would be decreased, and they would value themselves as persons at a level that was at least as equal to the value they place on their achievements.

Many people derive rewards for staying overweight. Maybe they get more attention from others regarding their helpless position—which can be interpreted that they are loved in spite of their weight. Their insecure husbands don't go into jealous rages. They are not expected to do as much, especially things they may be fearful of, like the woman whose husband would like to have her climb mountains with him if she could. Also, they may fear the loss of power. Size, with its implications of power, can be perceived or used as a means of intimidating people to control them or to get respect.

The reasons people don't do what they think they want to do when they know what to do go on and on. Each person can have a specific set of circumstances and background to point to. However, when all is examined closely, it usually comes down to the basics of fear and reward, which may be the same thing. People are usually afraid of losing something they have (i.e., a marriage) or of not getting something they want (i.e., perfection). Without taking the risk of facing our fears, we don't change in the way we perceive ourselves, helpless against food.

Unlike Mr. B., Louise has come to feel that it is more painful to stay the way she is than it will be to face her fears and change. By changing, she has a chance that her life may improve. We each have to make these hard decisions, take the risks, and try again and again until we reach our goals. Things will only get worse if we avoid facing our fears.

There are aspects of Louise in all of us that are even harder to change, because we are not consciously aware of them. Smells, for example, are our strongest memories and are tied to desires and fears, oftentimes without our even knowing when they are affecting us. When a person wants to lose weight on a conscious level, but has strong associations of food smells that bring back positive memories and comforting feelings of family, security and love, it is difficult to turn away from those foods, even though they may be fattening and unhealthy.

Associations between food smells, love, and security are more than just memories and desires, they become part of our subconscious beliefs and are capable of shaping and distorting our perceptions. If beliefs of this kind are buried deeply, they become very inaccessible and resistant to change. If we do not know what we subconsciously believe, we are likely to make choices on the basis of those beliefs without knowing it, causing us to do some illogical, contradictory and self-defeating things.

If we do try to change outwardly and it goes against our subconscious beliefs, great internal conflict and stress will follow. We are then struggling with two motives: 1) to make cognitive, logical decisions and act responsively to apparent needs; and 2) to avoid aspects of reality that threaten the subconscious beliefs to which we cling. Psychotherapy can uncover what we don't feel safe about letting out. Self-hypnosis can help us to feel safe about letting out deeper beliefs. This is like mastery: a self-determined discipline we practice until we love our skill and the self-efficacy that come with it.

The following chapter will be helpful in identifying your beliefs and values, and revealing how they are supported by the decisions you make. Nothing, however, will be as helpful as experiencing yourself behaving in ways in which you can trust yourself. When you trust yourself, your hidden beliefs are released easily.

Chapter 4

EMOTIONAL EATING, TOUCHING AND SEX

Hugs from the Refrigerator

*W*hen *Louise made her tenth trip to the refrigerator during an evening at home,* she usually wasn't thinking, "I'm feeling stressed, and I'm going to have a little snack to help me feel better for a few minutes." She initiated each trip in a mechanical, non-thinking manner. At times she would notice her frustration as she stood with the refrigerator door open, looking for some vague something that wasn't there twenty minutes ago and still wasn't there, wondering what it could be. Like millions of other Americans who do the same thing each day, Louise was bored (anxious, really) waiting for something to happen to stimulate her when she had no clear direction. Something that would bring purpose, value, pleasure, excitement, joy or peace to her life. With Louise, it could just as easily have been anger, fear, sadness, sexual tension, loneliness, or the lack of loving intimacy in her life that inspired those snack trips.

Food is sensual, evoking a feeling similar to that of being touched or hugged; so, therefore, it is comforting. It is also known that just tasting certain kinds of food—especially sweets, fats and carbohydrates—triggers a neuro-chemical reaction in the brain that almost instantly brings up feelings of pleasure, soothing comfort, and, at the very least, a distraction from the concerns of the day.

When she was at her weight loss group or in my office, Louise could clearly recognize the pattern and see the ease with which she had developed the habit of eating in response to her emotions. She could see she was using hugs from the refrigerator in an attempt to fulfill many emotional and physical needs. This is not surprising, considering food is a natural tranquilizer and a pleasurable distraction.

In this country, food is readily available to most of us at any time. Even those who are impoverished and whose pleasures might be limited often find pleasure in food. In fact, the food most available to lower income groups is often the most fattening. This may account for the higher incidence of weight problems among this group. Eating is easily justified since it is necessary to life. It is not usually perceived as harmful or anti-social, unlike other similar comforters such as alcohol, drugs or cigarettes. Being overweight may be looked down on, but eating excessively and inappropriately is encouraged and promoted in every segment of our society.

Louise was by no means alone in her behavior. A minimum of 85 percent of the overweight people I have worked with over the years could be regarded as emotional eaters: people who eat to fulfill other-than-nutritional needs. How to change emotional eating into pleasurable, healthful eating is the challenge (see Chapter 7).

Self-Awareness: The Starting Point

Understanding how unclarified beliefs and values can be an imperceptible and on-going source of stress is extremely important to dealing with the big picture, as well as to the long-term success for change and weight loss and the short-term self-awareness. We ask, "Why am I going to the refrigerator for another hug, and how can I stop it?"

Getting started on the process and beginning to deal with day-to-day, hour-to-hour urges to eat inappropriately requires more self-awareness. It also takes practice to learn the skills to deal with these urges and to train ourselves to follow new behaviors. If they have not been part of our life before, exercise, meditation and ways of dealing with our emotions and stress will take time to acquire. We need to be patient, not only with the learning about but also with the changing of ourselves.

Louise was very quick to catch on to the process of self-change I'm about to explain, but she was very slow to or apply her insights. She knew, for example, about what is commonly referred to as *self-talk*. She was aware of *imagery* (creating mental pictures), and she certainly could understand why it would be useful to be able to accurately monitor her feelings at any given moment. Louise also knew how to access and utilize these emotional factors. When at last she did decide this process was important enough to work, monitoring her self-talk, imagery, emotions and feelings soon became a part of her consciousness—developing into an on-going awareness as she needed it. The functional ability to balance and/or utilize her emotions and intellect to her own best advantage helped her to make choices that worked without a struggle.

Let Go of Control!

I wish to state clearly that the intent is never to *"control"* your emotions, but rather to utilize them by learning to find a *"harmony"* between the emotions you create in your mind and the physical needs of your body. Control is stressful. Control, like containing, forcing, or straining, only fatigues you. If you attempt to *control* your diet, you create a struggle between your will (intellectual resolve) and your emotional desires. The longer the struggle goes on, the more you tire. The desire to have what you emotionally want quickly exhausts your resistance and you give in to the urge to eat unhealthily.

Harmony is a relaxed, easy, flowing state that brings usable energy—moving you in the direction of what is a natural, healthful response to your body, mind, and spiritual needs. It is a state of homeostasis, or balance—and it is the opposite of excess or extreme.

For the most part, feelings (emotions) are generated from our thoughts, images, past experiences, and behaviors in response to our senses. Emotions are not something that just mysteriously grab us, nor are they only the result of things that happen to us or around us. Moreover, I believe we can create the emotions we choose to create by using our ability to speak to ourselves and by utilizing mental images, projecting into the future, reflecting on the past, and weighing these factors against our perceived beliefs of our own ability to deal effectively with the situations and circumstances (imagined or real) which we are facing.

Check in with Yourself

To deal with ourselves effectively (to choose to be fat or thin), it is very important to be aware of what we feel at the time we feel it. As young children, we start to learn to suppress our awareness of our feelings because it seems to be socially expedient, and we begin to realize that simply responding to our every stimulus with total abandonment isn't especially feasible, useful or considerate. Nevertheless, disconnecting ourselves from our emotional needs as adults in order to appear bright, quick, and poised, is too big of a price to pay.

Knowing what you are feeling (especially when your feelings are mild and not obvious) at the time you feel it, gives you better choices as to how your feelings will best fit together with your intellectual judgment. When you have achieved a balance between your feelings and intellect, you will find yourself behaving in ways that will work to your benefit.

Think of a scale, with your emotions on one side and your intellect on the other. It is important to keep them in balance. For example, when you are very focused on finding the solution to a math problem, and you are not thinking about passing or failing the test, you have your best chance of figuring out the problems. But if you start to wonder or worry if you'll get it right, or if you will pass or fail the test, your emotions interfere with your intellect, and your chances for failure increase. On another occasion, you may be very turned on to a developing sexual encounter when your partner asks a question of an analytical nature. Even if the discussion is only very brief, figuring out the answer will result in the loss of the sexual feelings you had moments before.

Although you may never experience a complete absence of either emotion or intellect, the more you have of one, the less you will have of the other. The ideal, of course, would be to reach a balance.

Gradually redeveloping your ability to always be in touch with even your most mild feelings is very simple—it only takes practice. Ask yourself as many times each day as you can think of it, "what am I feeling?" Listen to your body, and it will tell you. This should only take a split second. Practice it now!

If you just tried to analyze your feelings, you missed the point. You create your feelings in your head, and you experience them in your body. You may remember the physical sensations you experienced when you came close to having a car accident. Your heart may have raced, your stomach turned over, muscles tightened, etc. Your body reacts to less threatening situations in the same, although milder, way. These mild feelings are the feelings we have learned to ignore.

Think of your body as a barometer. When your feelings are around your ankles, they are very mild. As they build to your knees, your legs may feel rubbery. By the time they reach your stomach, you have indigestion. At your chest, you have chest pains or rapid heart beats. At your mouth, your breath is short or you jumble your words. After your emotions build past your eyes, you are blinded to them, and you are apt to do or say something you will regret later.

Monitoring your emotions gives you some of the awareness you need to keep them in harmony with your logic or intellect. Practicing a hundred times each day need not interfere with whatever else you may be doing. If you don't sense your emotions in the recommended split second, come back to them again later. It will soon become natural and easy and require no special effort. Remember, you always have more than one feeling at any given moment. Mixed emotions (a variety of feelings) are not necessarily contrary in making your decisions. For example, excitement may occur together with fear. The more powerful of these feelings may be fear, and it may hold the most potential for change as well. For, if we embrace our fears we can resolve them and as a result, our self-image grows along with our confidence to face our fears tomorrow.

Back to Louise

Louise walked to her car after a visit to the doctor. He had been late, the examination of her back had been painful, and she had a headache. If she didn't hurry, she would not have time for supper, or would be late for her group meeting, or both. The air out in the parking lot was hot, as only September in Arizona can be, and as she approached her car she saw one of the tires was flat. It was rush-hour, she was in the middle of downtown where everything closed by six o'clock, and it would be dark in an hour. It was not a safe place to be.

Her heart sank into her stomach the moment she noticed the problem. In that blink of a moment, she imagined herself unable to locate a towing service or paying a big fee for one; and trying to fix the tire herself with her dislocated disk, in dress clothes, in 105-degree heat. She could not call her husband for help, as he was on patrol duty in another part of town. She pictured herself stranded in the parking lot after dark, being robbed or raped, and these images brought on a feeling of panic.

The point is, it only took a split second for Louise to become extremely upset. It wasn't the flat tire that made her upset, *it was what she told herself about the tire*. Our minds are faster than any computer in a situation like this. We talk to ourself and picture in our minds all of the horrible consequences that could result from the circumstances that we find ourselves in.

We talk to ourselves constantly, although we are often not consciously aware of doing so. We ask questions of ourselves and give answers or debate outcomes. Sometimes we talk to ourselves out loud—and to me, that only means we can hear ourselves better. What we do with this self-talk can vary a great deal. One thing is certain: self-talk contributes a great deal to creating one's mood from moment-to-moment. We talk ourselves up or down or into a mellow state. We talk ourselves into or out of decisions and, in my opinion, we even talk ourselves into love. Talking to ourselves is an on-going process to which we pay far too little attention.

When Louise was in the doctor's office, she was not feeling well, but not yet knowing anything about her flat tire, she could still see a way of handling all her concerns of the day. Once she had awareness of the tire, it all fell apart. Her self-talk raced ahead, and panic, depression, and frustration all set in at the same time. All of her earlier resolutions about how to deal with her concerns were wiped out.

As it turned out, the husband of one of the nurses was stopping for his wife in his pickup truck and had Louise's spare onto her car in a matter of minutes. Louise laughed about it in her support group that evening. She also realized then that her headache and backache were forgotten in her anxiety over the situation she found herself in the doctor's parking lot. The point is, Louise had a choice about her emotional response to the whole predicament. She could have laughed at the final straw to a bad day and gone back into the office for help, or she could do what she did and create a feeling of panic. Many things could and did influence her feelings, but she also had clear choices about how she added to or detracted from those other emotional influences.

Creating Mental Pictures

In addition to the self-talk that had gone on in Louise's head, she also created mental pictures (imagery and fantasies) which contributed greatly to the resulting feelings. She saw (projected with mental pictures) all of the possible negative outcomes of her situation. She saw herself dirty, in pain, paying for a tow truck, getting attacked, being late, hungry, etc. These pictures added a sort of reality to her words that exacerbated her emotions tenfold. The power of mental pictures is so great that it is hard to estimate the extent of their effect. Use mental pictures to recall some of your more wonderful and awful dreams. Hopefully, we do not overlook these waking fantasies and their relationship to emotions, eating, and weight.

Allow yourself to imagine that you're in your kitchen. You walk to the refrigerator and open it. There, in front of you, is the biggest, most perfect, beautiful lemon you have ever seen. It is flawless. You take it out, and in the warmth of the room, moisture condenses on the cool lemon, and little rivulets of water start to pool in your hand. You take the lemon to your counter and cut it into wedges. You pick up the largest wedge and deeply inhale its fragrance. You can see the little membrane is just bursting with juice. Just by looking at it and smelling it you can already taste it, and you open your mouth wide and bite fully into the lemon wedge.

If you have been following along with pictures in your mind, the muscles in your throat contracted, and you puckered or salivated. This picture story demonstrates how powerful mental pictures are in creating emotions. Feelings are created by mental pictures about most everything we worry about or look forward to. You can use your mental pictures for or against yourself. If you are going to utilize your mental pictures to your advantage, again, it will be as a result of practice and learned skill.

Start by picturing some of your favorite places. Places where you feel safe and comfortable. These can be places you have experienced or places you've created only in your imagination, just so you find pleasure in them and want to return to them. Practice frequently by getting into the details of the scenery, the clarity of the picture, and bringing your senses into it. For example, see yourself at the beach. The temperature is ideal, and you see yourself seated in the sand. You can feel the warmth of the sun on your body and the cool breeze on your skin, and you can smell the sea water. You feel the soft sand underneath you, and you pick up a handful of warm sand and notice the grains of sand separate and run through your fingers. Only a few people are on the beach, and the scene is very peaceful to you. You notice the sharp bright colors of the swim suits, the sizes of the bodies, the ages of the people, the shells and seaweed on the shore, and the sound of the waves as they break against some large rocks. The laughter of the children playing encourages feelings of how good the water would feel. This becomes a vivid picture, full of details and brings your senses into play.

The more you practice mental imagery, the more you can use your fantasies and dreams to your advantage.

Putting It Together

By monitoring your emotions, self-talk, and mental pictures, you will find you will be better able to feel the calm and harmony within yourself and you will develop confidence about your ability to deal with the situations of your life.

Clarifying beliefs and values and making decisions that are consistent with them, monitoring emotions, using positive self-talk and mental pictures are all basic steps we can take toward self-directed change over the long term, and of day-to-day emotions and behavior in the short term. Once you have developed the ability to utilize these abilities constructively, other parts of your life will come together. Your self-esteem will rise, and the other traits you share with "the fat personality" will be modified.

You will never be able to remove all stress from your life, but the incidents of distress that lead you to the refrigerator will decrease, and you will handle them in a very different, self-enhancing manner.

Self-esteem needs are also met (e.g., knowing what you believe, value, and feel; making decisions that fit; and being responsible for your feelings and thus your behavior). You must give yourself this positive time, attention, and energy, just as you must meet your basic human needs for sex and touching.

Touching

Touching is now known to be a necessary element to promote human growth and development, as well as to promote a healthy immune system. Volumes have been written describing the statistical, experimental, and clinical research that has been done on the subject of touching. However, it is still unusual to find a question on a medical history or stress assessment questionnaire about touching, which may testify as to how uncomfortable our society is with the subject. It is a sad and common reality that the only time some people are touched is by paying for it, such as by the chiropractor, the hair dresser, or a professional masseuse. Even many health practitioners, such as doctors, nurses, or counselors who know the healing power of touch are afraid to touch or hug their clients or patients because, in our modern-day, distrustful, litigious society, they may be misunderstood and sued for making improper advances. Also, the health practitioners may be so up-tight about being touched themselves, that they rationalize and justify their avoidance of this important human need.

After the honeymoon period of marriage wears off, husband and wife frequently only touch during sexual contact or in parting or arriving home. Children, all too often, are deprived of parental touch after reaching adolescence. This is unfortunate. Touching is a part of communication. It is a means of being reassured that we are cared for and loved. It can provide us with a sense of security and well-being that assures us in ways words can't always do. It is easy to understand how, in a critical, competitive society such as ours, true intimacy is very hard to come by. It may seem safer to get our hugs from the refrigerator. Because we reserve touching for such special occasions, we lose awareness of its greater value and forget its importance and possible connection to the needs in our day-to-day lives.

With the prejudice found in this society against being overweight (even among overweight people themselves), and the premium that is put on the trim body, along with the other previously mentioned factors of social discrimination, embarrassment, and public attitudes, is it any wonder that overweight people frequently develop an aversion to being touched? In fact, some of the overweight people I've met who need touching the most, fear it to the point of being phobic about it. The longer we avoid that which we need and fear, the greater the chance we will become paranoid about it. A person who likes himself or herself for the person he or she is and not just for their performance will be comfortable with touching and intimacy and automatically accept and initiate it as a natural valued experience. Real hugs can replace the hugs from the refrigerator very effectively.

Clearly, Louise was not getting enough touching at home. This lack not only contributed to her weight problem, but also to becoming involved in extramarital affairs, separation from her husband, and possible divorce. The possible correlation between eating, weight gain, touching and sex are not always recognized.

Sex and Overeating

Food is very sensual—i.e., it appeals to the senses—as is sexual activity. Both eating and engaging in sex can have a temporary calming effect. Therefore, it is easy to see how the one may be substituted for the other and the substitution never noticed. The healthy human body prepares itself many times each day for a sexual encounter. Even though age has a bearing on frequency, the biological phenomenon can last throughout our lives, baring illness, excessive stress or fatigue. If we seldom respond to our libidinous drive, a sexual tension builds up which needs some outlet. Because we have commonly cut ourselves off from our milder feelings as a result of our social fears, stigmas, and competitive drives for security and approval, recognizing or attending to our sexual needs tends to take a low priority on our motivation and value scale. It can be easy to find yourself haunting the refrigerator for snack food a hundred times over and never make the connection between your sexual needs and the unexplained, unquenchable appetite.

The only times I've seen people recognize some relationship between sex and eating is when the exchange had gone to an extreme; where intercourse had stopped completely for a long period of time, and eating rituals had become more and more elaborate and exotic, evolving into a clear sexual medium between partners. This is well depicted in the movie, *The Loved Ones,* when the character Joy Boy, played by Rod Stieger, has a vicarious, incestuous relationship with his morbidly obese mother.

Hugs from the refrigerator can be used as a substitute for unmet sexual needs; they also may offer the comforting we miss from the lack of loving relationships. Biologically, mentally and sociologically, we have sexual drives. When these drives go unfulfilled, it is easy and convenient to subconsciously provide for our needs with food—sensual food—and not be aware of what we are doing, or why.

Periodically, discuss your sexual needs with a trusted person (maybe even your spouse) to become more self-aware. When an acceptable sexual partner is not available, auto-eroticism is normal and provides for sexual release in a manner more healthful than inappropriate eating.

Chapter 5

THE BASE FOR CHANGE

Beliefs, Values, Decisions and Self-Esteem

*L*ike *almost all the people I've seen over the years, Louise was at a loss* when I asked the question, "what is your philosophy of life"? No matter what the person's station in life, age, I.Q., profession, or income level, I have yet to get more than a flip or rote answer to my question. It isn't that people don't have a set of beliefs, it is more that they have never done "an analysis of the grounds of and concepts expressing fundamental beliefs; an overall vision of or attitude toward life and the purpose of life."

As a young student working my way through college, I remember being asked on employment forms about my philosophy of life. At that time, it seemed irrelevant, and I would write down whatever came into my mind just to get it out of the way. Now, after facilitating hundreds of people to change, I realize that recognizing and defining one's philosophy of life (belief system) is essential in order for intrinsic change to occur. To me, it is like wanting to go on a trip to a specific destination: if I don't know where I am starting from, it is awfully hard to determine the direction in which I must travel. Similarly, if I do not know who I am, how can I even know who I want to be? Most clients are able to give me a chronology of their life, but they aren't clear about who they are as a person. Often, it is the lack of value they have for themselves as a person that is a major part of the problem.

Like Louise, everyone has been so busy trying to live up to what they imagine others expect of them that they do not have time to concern themselves with who they are. Instead, they do not consider much beyond simply a matter of how to get on with the next task to reach the next goal. To operate otherwise seems frivolous and produces guilt. In the case of Louise, for example, and her sense of low self-worth, taking the time to nurture her own well-being would mean taking away time from her external focus (the caretaker/people-pleaser) and this would threaten her security. As a result, she just keeps plowing ahead, the same way she always has, not knowing why or if it fits with her beliefs or not.

Part of my convictions are that everything we do, think, and feel comes out of our beliefs directly or indirectly. Our beliefs influence every aspect of our life every minute of every day we are alive. They are the basis for our motivation to do, or not to do, anything. If part of what I believe is that my performance is my only true value or worth in life, then I believe that if I can't do many things—or even one thing—I'm apt to be rejected (not loved). Therefore, it would be easy for me to become a perfectionist and not know why. However, each of us don't have just one belief, we have many—a set, or system of beliefs about almost everything we've encountered. Even if I am not sure what I believe, if I state that, then it becomes my belief. We don't escape our beliefs, but we may not be aware of them.

Think of yourself as a loan manager at a bank. With your signature alone, you are authorized to lend $50,000 of the bank's money. One of your many beliefs may be that humans are basically evil or basically good, or your belief may be that humans simply have the potential to be good or evil. No matter what you believe in this instance, you can see that it will clearly affect the way you do (or don't) give out loans. Although with the approach of each new loan applicant you may not be consciously thinking about your belief that people are either good or evil, your decision undoubtedly will be influenced by this basic belief. Of course, even if you are not a bank loan manager, it is clearly useful to know your beliefs when planning to change your life-style.

You can see how simply one belief can have a potentially big effect on our actions and decisions. Imagine, then, how powerful all of your beliefs together are in determining your every thought, behavior, and feeling.

Out of our beliefs come what we consider to be the meaning and purpose of our life. The better we understand what we consider to be the meaning and purpose of our life, the better we can handle the difficulties life hands us. Once you are able to understand why you are struggling with something, you will be able to endure adversity and you will feel better about doing it.

A good illustration of this is made in Viktor Frankl's book, *Man's Search for Meaning*, which describes the desperate experience of prisoners in a Nazi death camp. Many of those who could not identify a reason to live or could not name anything to make continuing the struggle worthwhile— e.g., for family, to help others, or even for revenge—experienced intense despair, gave up and died. Others who were able to identify or discover a meaning and purpose for living, even under such horrible conditions, made it through, often enduring greater hardships than those who died. What sustained them was largely their ability to identify that their life had meaning. No matter how difficult the circumstance, "changing" the meaning can get us through.

It is my conviction that when our beliefs are not clear to us, we experience what appears to be a void or empty space inside ourselves. It is an unknown, and unknowns frighten us. When our beliefs, like the value priorities which follow from them, are not clear to us, they are unknowns and this produces on-going, low level anxiety. Over time, the discomfort becomes almost imperceptible. Our state of mild anxiety becomes so familiar, it seems normal or usual. To suddenly feel fully calm might even seem strange or even frightening.

On-going, low level anxiety, unlike the anxiety we experience when we almost have a car accident, wears us down. Our immune system weakens, making us more subject to illnesses, and we are more vulnerable to experiencing distress from vicissitudes of daily life. We react to stressors more often, more quickly and more strongly, and our reactions last longer when we have continuous, low level anxiety. Of course, more emotion means more need for comfort from that sensual nemesis: food. That is, more hugs from the refrigerator.

When you think about your philosophy of life, open your mind and contemplate what is true for all people that have ever lived or ever might live. Being able to identify your philosophy of life will go a long way toward reducing anxiety by building confidence and filling up the internal void. It will also get you started on clarifying your value priorities, as they are built upon your beliefs.

Use the following "philosophy-of-life organizer" to gain some insight into yourself. Plan to take your time, be patient, and follow the steps in order to learn more about the base your life is built upon.

YOUR PHILOSOPHY-OF-LIFE ORGANIZER

Figuring out a philosophy of life (i.e., set of beliefs) requires time, reading, observing, experiencing, and continual discussion. You will be writing and rewriting until you it is clear to you. Some people make the mistake of assuming that this task can be done off the top of their heads in five minutes. If that's the time they give it, that's exactly how deep, meaningful, lasting, and valuable it will be to them.

In reality, there is no set way to uncover your philosophy of life, and the project will never be completely finished. However, by establishing a base point, each person can be on top of his or her beliefs/values and then attune to gradual changes that occur as life is experienced. We will be much more sure of who we are, which is invaluable in reaching our goals. Consider the following guide to help illuminate your beliefs.

What are your beliefs for people, in general? Which of the beliefs you have for all people fit in with your beliefs about yourself? Go through the list below to determine what you believe to be true for every one else. Then, try to define your personal beliefs. Use a separate paper and change and add material until you feel comfortable and complete with your answers.

Remember, this list is only to stimulate your own thoughts and ideas. You are always in a state of becoming. What you are becoming has a great deal to do with your beliefs. You are free to choose that for which you can like yourself.

What I believe is true for all humans, forever and always:	What I believe is true for me:
We have free choice (i.e., to be fat or thin).	I choose to be _____.
Purpose and meaning are essential to inner peace, happiness and endurance.	My purpose and meaning in life come from _____.
We each determine our own truth.	I have faith in _____.
Movement (change) is a constant part of life (including living, growing and even dying).	The direction for my life today and tomorrow is _____.
Love is the most powerful force.	My ability to love is _____.
Questions, challenges and problems are essential to a positive self-image.	The questions, challenges and problems I give priority to are: _____.
Humans have the potential to be good or evil and are free to determine what is good or evil.	Basically my life is: _____.
All things are connected; i.e., all things can lead to something better.	My ability to function in harmony with other things and grow from discord is _____.
All people are unique or special and yet them same.	My special uniqueness is _____.
Reality and illusion can be the same.	What I imagine can lead me to _____.
Self-identity comes from observation, comparison, decision and responses to experiences.	My self-identity will develop _____.
Balance or centeredness brings out human potentials.	My stability comes from _____.
Individual, basic drives are often misinterpreted or ignored.	My value priorities are: _____.

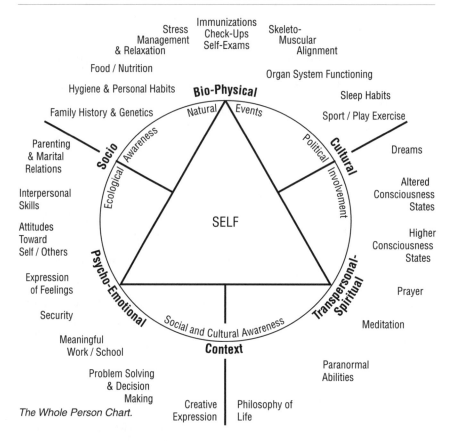

Immunizations
Stress · Check-Ups · Skeleto-
Management · Self-Exams · Muscular
& Relaxation · Alignment

Food / Nutrition

Hygiene & Personal Habits · **Bio-Physical** · Organ System Functioning

Family History & Genetics · Natural / Events · Sleep Habits

Socio · *Awareness* · *Political Involvement* · *Cultural* · Sport / Play Exercise

Parenting & Marital Relations · Dreams

Interpersonal Skills · *Ecological* · Altered Consciousness States

Attitudes Toward Self / Others · SELF · Higher Consciousness States

Expression of Feelings · *Psycho-Emotional* · *Transpersonal-Spiritual* · Prayer

Security · Meditation

Meaningful Work / School · *Social and Cultural Awareness* · **Context**

Problem Solving & Decision Making · Paranormal Abilities

The Whole Person Chart. · Creative Expression · Philosophy of Life

If you complete those sentences about your personal beliefs (note: you will need more space than has been provided!) and adjust or accept the beliefs you have about all people until you are comfortable with them, then you are ready to start monitoring your readings, conversations, observations, etc. Question your beliefs as you complete the exercise and adjust each new draft until you run out of new questions and thoughts.

Then write your final draft, and reread it until you can verbalize it without the aid of what you have written down. Gradually, you will come to the point that you will notice changes in your beliefs as they are happening.

Even if you don't incorporate any of the other self-enhancement suggestions offered in this book, if you really do clarify your own beliefs in the manner described it will have a major, positive impact upon your life.

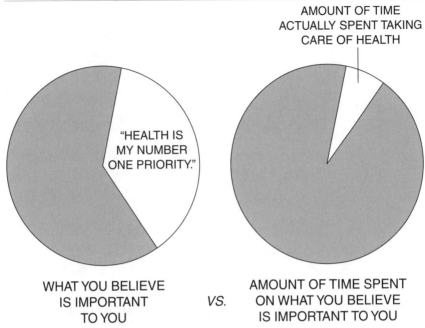

Your Value Priorities.

You will be calmer, more thoughtful, more decisive, more understanding, more fulfilled, more integrated, more authentic, and more successful.

YOUR VALUE PRIORITIES

Knowing what you value and how your values rank in priority is the second step towards achieving the self-awareness needed for self-directed change. Clarifying your values will take time, effort, and a good deal of reevaluation. If your interest and belief in these priorities is not there; or if identifying, categorizing, and establishing their order of importance is not a high priority for you, complete the process another time. Just going through the motions to say you have completed the task will be of little value to your change process.

Think in terms of writing three to six drafts before you are comfortable with knowing what is important to you. Ideally, between drafts there will be a great deal of thought and discussion with those who know you well, and observation and dissecting of all of aspects of your life (see the Whole Person Chart, previous page). As illustrated in the two pie charts above

(Your Value Priorities), you can compare what you believe is most important to you to the manner in which you actually use your time. Is there a discrepancy, or are they equal? A visual of the past can show how you have changed, and a chart of the future shows your plans to change. If you can, reflect back with people who know what you have done, for this helps you to value the changes you've made. It also helps to follow this reflection on your past with a projection of the rest of your life in an effort to imagine changing needs and activities before finalizing your values.

No matter how "perfect" your priority list is, time and experience will require you to question your values and modification will be likely. However, once your values are a part of your consciousness, you will notice any changes as you make them. The closer you come to living by your own value priorities, the more you will trust yourself, and the less you will have doubts about what you can or can't do.

Remember, your beliefs are the base upon which your values are built. Like beliefs, if your value structure is unclear to you, you may create an almost imperceptible anxiety within yourself. If you continually choose lesser values over your more important values, you may not even notice until you are paying a price you'd rather not pay.

In other words, if you commonly favor value number 20 over value number 2 and you aren't aware of it, you will find it hard to relax, to like and to trust yourself.

Being aware of ourselves includes being aware of what we believe life is about, and the order of importance with which we hold these ideas, people, property, and/or experiences. Start with the most important things (other than life itself) and work down to at least value number 20. Begin by asking: if you had to give up everything in your life except one thing, what would that be? Perhaps the answer is your children, or maybe it is your parents, your spouse, your career, your health, your religion, etc... Whatever it is, that is your first value priority. Keep going until you have identified your top 20 priorities. You'll notice before you finish that your priorities all overlap. For instance, perhaps value #1 is your health, and value #2 your children. However, to some degree, your health determines what you are able to give to your children, and there is overlap.

If you are wise, you will take your time, rethink your choices and go over our list again and again. You have already changed your value priorities many times in your life. Now you want to have them clear to you form day to day, knowing when and why they change. This will help you to be emotionally stronger and better able to establish direction in your life—even to find meaning and purpose in what you are doing with your life. Most of all, this knowledge will enable you to make better decisions—decisions you make every day, all day, from the time you become conscious each morning until you fall asleep each night. Our lives are a continuing series of decisions, such as: *Do you believe what you are reading here? Will you complete the task? When will you do it? And, in what manner will you do it?*

Not only are we constantly deciding about something, each decision we make affects our self-image. When our decisions are in keeping with our values, we like ourselves better, we trust ourselves more, and we fear our decisions less. We don't have to be perfect and, therefore, we come much closer to our potential to be happy, loving, insightful, creative, kind, giving, bright and physically healthy—and yes, maybe even to be more successful. With your beliefs and value priorities clear in your mind, monitoring the decisions that lead to your improved self-image will go smoothly.

MY VALUE PRIORITIES

(Start with what is most important to you and work down.)

1. _____

2. _____

3. _____

4. _____

5. _____

6. _____

7. _____

8. _____

9. _____

10. _____

11. _____

12. _____

13. _____

14. _____

15. _____

16. _____

17. _____

18. _____

19. _____

20. _____

21. _____

22. _____

23. _____

24. _____

25. _____

DECISIONS

Louise was keenly aware of which foods were most healthful and least fattening, but routinely she would choose fattening foods as she went through her choices at restaurants, the grocery store, and while holding open the door of her refrigerator. When you imagine how many times she made these choices over the years, even after she became aware of the truth about her choices and knew that one of her highest value priorities "should" be her health, you can imagine how her view of herself was being chipped away at every time she ate fattening, unhealthy food. The message to herself was, "Louise, you can't trust yourself, and your own life isn't as important as all the people you care for." The occasions on which she would make healthful choices, of course, would somewhat balance out the self-defeating choices, so the whole process became like a batting average. The more times she went to the "plate," the harder it was to change her average. When Louise's choices were predominantly self-defeating (against her health/weight values) her self-image dropped more than it was raised. Considering all the other choices (decisions) in her life that could be either aligned with or in opposition to her own beliefs or value priorities, you can see how her total self-image moved up and down.

What we witness ourselves doing as a result of our decisions becomes what we believe to be true about who we are. Again, for Louise to change a view she held about herself took time—it was gradual and involved most aspects of her life. She had to be more sensitive and self-aware so she could realize new self-enhancing choices. Most of all, to turn around her self-image, she had to be patiently brave, calling upon her courage, in spite of her own poor image of herself, to face the hard decisions, risk failure, and do it over and over until the changes created a new and improved view of herself that she believed.

Beliefs, values, and decisions are the basis for self-change and interact with all the things you might do to achieve the trim body you seek. A number of the other basic things on which you will test your beliefs, values, and decisions will be covered in the next chapter. Remember, you don't have to change everything all at once. In fact, please do not try. Go slowly, and it will happen. All parts of "the whole you" are important, and the more you bring them together, the faster your desires will be attained.

Books and videotapes such as Joseph Campbell's *The Power of Myth* and *The Book of Questions* may help you to get started identifying your beliefs and values. Sometimes reading them before trying to clarify your own beliefs can be helpful. However, it is not necessary to read them to complete the exercise.

Chapter 6

DE-STRESSING DISTRESS

S *tress, the socio-emotional behaviors that result from stress, and the* lack of coping or adjustment skills are the primary cornerstones of my wellness theory of weight gain/loss.

Emotional eating patterns vary a great deal within any group of people. Some individuals may be unable to eat if they are experiencing any amount of stress, while others may eat more when their stress levels are escalated. This latter was the case with Louise. Depression, loneliness, sorrow, joy, or excitement at a high or low intensity usually meant she would eat more.

Fear and anxiety are by far the emotions most commonly responsible for sending people to the refrigerator for a hug. Whenever a person perceives a threat to his or her security, desires, needs, or wants, he or she is apt to exhibit some type of physical and/or emotional response that could be classified as stress. When it is functioning well, our neurochemical system reacts to all changes in our environment with some degree of stress, but it is when we consciously perceive a change or possible change and we question or doubt our ability to cope that our stress symptoms appear and our ability to function at our best is impaired.

Even positive emotions such as excitement, happiness, or joy can be stressful. Your body does not distinguish between the types of emotions you are experiencing, only the degree of intensity. Physical injury or illness produces stress, as does excessive fatigue, obesity, or the trauma of exerting vast reserves of energy. In all these instances, your body and mind prepare to defend themselves, balance themselves, or remove you from the situation.

Stress, then, is your physical/mental (body/mind) reactions to real or imagined environmental changes and the perceived threat to your survival or equilibrium. Your senses bring you messages, your brain measures them, your mind determines if you can handle them, and your body experiences *usable stress* (for example, superior recall of rehearsed lines while performing on stage), *manageable stress* (such as controlled but unimaginative job interview responses) or *distress* (for example, deliberate binges).

SYMPTOMS OF STRESS AND DISTRESS

Remember, some symptoms of stress are too slight to be noticed. Some symptoms we have either disconnected ourselves from or have suppressed because we mistakenly think they interfere with the way we want to be perceived by others. Some symptoms are noticed more by others than ourselves. Some symptoms demand that we take notice. These latter are the ones we are most familiar with. Many times while they are being measured for stress levels, biofeedback clients have told me they felt relaxed (and they believed it) when the feedback clearly reported fairly high levels of stress. Many of us have become very skilled at blocking our own responses.

There are nearly as many symptoms as there are causes. The following are some typical causes of stress:

- Illness—anything from allergies to cancer
- Disordered thinking
- Hypertension
- Excessive drinking
- Difficulty in sleeping or relaxing
- Speech impairments
- Poor concentration
- Nervous tics
- Hyperactive behavior/speech
- Lack of joy found in entertainment

- Loss of sense of humor

- Low sexual interest or impotence

- Vision problems

- Muscle/structural problems

- Rapid heart/pulse/breathing

- Paralysis

- Loss of energy

- Short temper

- Loss of interest in old pleasures

- Frequent withdrawal from usual activities.

SOURCES OF STRESS

Causes of stress are as many as the many changes that occur in our lives. Any change perceived by our senses or imagined by our mind can be stressful. Some stress is generalized, some is very specific. Some stress is learned and becomes a conditioned response; some comes through trauma or shock. Pollution, the economy, traffic congestion, war, crime, jobs, unemployment (or the threat of it), romance (or the lack of it), body image, injury, drinking, smoking, poor diet, children, or parents can be the start of an endless list of what are called *stressors*. What you believe about your environment and your ability to cope with it has everything to do with how you determine what will be usable stress, manageable stress or distress.

DISTRESS PREVENTION AND STRESS MANAGEMENT

Prevention and management of stress and distress are important for people who are seeking wellness as much or more than weight loss. The quality of your life—and the quality of the people who are in your life—are greatly enhanced by the practice of the following list of basic wellness habits. Once a "stress storm" is in progress, learning or utilizing these practices is of much less value—rather like installing the smoke detector during the fire. Think of these practices as adding to your life in terms of quality and achievements. The important aspects of stress management are:

1. *Self-awareness*

Become aware of the connection between what is happening in your mind and body in relationship to your environment. This is a natural ability which you can relearn simply by practicing listening to yourself and becoming aware of yourself until it becomes a habit that is done without conscious effort. Candid discussion and feedback from others who know you is also helpful.

2. *Exercise*

Establish a frequent (four or more times a week), varied routine that is safe, progressively more vigorous, and balanced (including stretching, contracting, and aerobic exercise), with satisfactory recovery time in between.

3. *Rest*

Take time for sufficient sleep (a full eight hours—which is more than most adults think they need), dreamwork and waking fantasy, and for calming practices, such as meditation.

4. *Nutrition*

Initiate healthful eating routines, which gradually reduce sugar, salt, and fat intake, with a wide, increased variety of whole grains, whole fruits and vegetables, beans, and a few seeds/nuts. Vitamin and mineral supplements are also recommended for those who insist on using weight loss diets and during periods of high stress.

5. *Support system*

Develop emotional, social, career, and physical support from organizations, personal beliefs, secure places, and friends and loved ones who appreciate you, nurture your development, and have their own healthful lifestyle, or at least are working on it.

6. *Calming activities*

Enjoy pursuits which add to your well-being and strengthen your resolve to change. We all must find our own calming activities. Putting my thoughts on paper is one of mine; walking with a special person or alone is another. For some people it's fishing; for others it could be art, music, gardening, etc.

7. *Environment*

Make sure your surroundings include clean air, full spectrum light, enough space, comfortable noise levels, pleasing colors, safe radiation and radon levels, and safe building materials and furnishings.

Ensuring that these factors are a part of the lifestyle you choose for yourself is important and will go a long way toward keeping a good deal of stress from becoming distress. It will even enable you to capitalize on useful stress. It isn't helpful to strain to be perfect in all of these areas, but simply try to give them priority when the choice is yours.

DE-STRESSING STRESS

The movement from stress to distress may be slowed, stopped or reversed simply by using the following intellectual analysis. If you have incorporated the prevention methods indicated above into your lifestyle, the following steps will be a quick, practical exercise for you:

1. *Acknowledge your feelings.*

Acknowledgement of your feelings means to be in touch with them and to admit *you* have developed them. Try not to let your ego get in the way. This is not a matter of lack of intelligence or any other flaw in you, but rather learned behavior which you can change through awareness.

2. *Identify your emotions.*

Know your emotions for what they are. Do they include anger, fear, hurt, frustration, joy, peace, love, sexiness, hate, calm, excitement, etc.? The more accurate you are in identifying your emotions, the more effectively you will be able to deal with them. Remember, you are likely to experience more than one emotion at any given moment.

3. *Determine the level of the feelings you are experiencing.*

Which feelings are slight? Which are strong? Are you only ill-at-ease, or are you about to lose what you think of as "control"?

4. *Ask, "What am I doing with these feelings?"*

Are you straining to make them go away? Are your self-talk and mental pictures building the feelings up, or toning them down? Are you pushing them into your subconscious? Are you examining them closely and dissipating them? You're the boss!

5. *Determine the source you are using to create your stress.*

Are you giving a conditioned response? Are you creating stress about something you worried about or predicted would happen? Is the source of your stress something new and confusing that you fear you may not be able to deal with? Is it something from within or from outside of yourself (for example, unexplained physical pain versus someone trying to sabotage you at work)? Are you projecting, reflecting, or dealing with the present time? Is your stress about survival (food, air, health)? Is it the unknown? What are the dynamics of your stress? It may take some intellectual detective work or analysis to determine the source you are using to create your stress, but engaging in the deductive process itself will reduce stress. Finding the root cause you've focused on can help you to understand why you've chosen to create the stress and will give you better options for dealing with it effectively.

6. *Express your feelings positively.*

Finding a positive expression for your feelings is the last step you will need in reducing stress if you have sincerely completed the first five steps. All of the steps mentioned above are part of an intellectual self-awareness, and, as your level intellectual reasoning increases, your emotional stimulation goes down. It's a matter of balance.

If, however, you have a residual amount of emotion to dissipate, express your feelings in ways that will not hurt you or others (nor cause others to defend themselves). Raise your voice or really yell. As long as you are not blaming others or putting them down, most people can deal with a little noise, and you will feel better. Expend physical energy. Run, jump up and down, hit *soft* things that you can't hurt and which can't hurt you. Look in the mirror and "sincerely" strain to look and feel as upset as you can (it becomes a paradox; the harder your try to look and feel upset, the harder it is to stay upset). Visualize or write in a letter you won't send that which would be self-defeating if you did it openly.

PRINCIPLES OF DE-STRESSING

The techniques you can use to de-stress yourself are almost as unlimited as those stressors you've acquired to stress yourself. Any techniques I am aware of tend to include all or most of the principles listed below. If any stress reduction technique is to have a good chance of being useful to you, the practice of it will be initiated by you, without pre-determined judgments, but rather with a mind open to possible outcomes. It will be practiced with great regularity, and it will be most helpful to you if it was created or modified by you to meet your special circumstances.

1. *Let down your defenses.*

Allow your mind to be quiet. Relax your muscles. Reduce the stimuli to your senses—sight, smell, taste, sound, hearing.

2. *Have a focus and keep it simple.*

Your focus can be external or internal. It can be an imagined object or a real object. Use one of your senses to focus on a movement, an object, a sound, a color, a smell, or a taste. Focus on one single thing, such as your breathing.

3. *Choose a safe place.*

It is important, especially at the start, to practice de-stressing activities where you feel sure you will encounter no interruptions, danger, or distractions. As you progress, you will be able to tolerate more stimuli. Build your confidence first.

4. *Try to have a rested mind and an empty stomach.*

An active stomach makes it hard for your mind to relax. Being tired and ready for sleep means you probably will fall asleep rather than practicing stress relief. You may not be consciously aware of your stress while you're sleeping, but you will have done nothing to eliminate it. It will be there when you wake up.

5. *Do not strain to relax.*

Straining to relax creates a paradox. Push, force, and strain to relax, and you'll become more tense. Strain to stay awake, and you fall asleep. The key to achieving relaxation is learning how to "let go."

6. *Be aware that the magic that will allow you to relax is inside.*

You hold the key to relaxing. To use it the key you must practice before the storm. External, quick fixes are temporary, habit forming, dangerous, lower your opinion of yourself, and end up creating more stress. The sooner you quit looking for the magic outside, the sooner you will find it inside.

7. *Find your harmony button.*

The relaxation technique that is most likely to work for you is the one that appeals to you most; i.e., the one you believe in. This is the one you are most apt to practice to the point that you are able to shorten the process so that a single "cue," such as a certain word, sound, movement, image, or color, is all you need to slip into a relaxed, harmonious state.

When you are in the process of learning a relaxation technique, remember, you are learning far more than the technique, and you are after more than the ability to relax. You are attempting to change your image of yourself by demonstrating to yourself your willingness to consistently give yourself the time and energy you need to follow through on your commitment to yourself—even when you don't feel like practicing and when requests from people you care about could easily take you away from it. If you consistently (but not rigidly) nurture your own need in this manner over a meaningfully long period of time, you will not only master the task, but you will also increase your self-esteem, self-worth, self-confidence, and self-trust. This all translates into less doubt about whether you will or won't eat and exercise in a healthful manner.

The rate at which each person develops mastery of any of the methods or techniques suggested in this chapter depends on their personal history and the circumstances in which they work, play, and live. Some people are afraid to relax. To them, relaxing feels like loss of control. Others get excited about the possibility of relaxing. Some doubt themselves so much they give up. And some pick it up quickly, simply by permitting it to happen.

The following techniques are but a small representation of the hundreds that are known to facilitate relaxation. However, almost everyone will be able to find at least one acceptable technique on the list. Or, feel free to modify or create your own. In fact, the ones you come up with will be the ones that you are most apt to use, value, and practice the longest. Most of these methods are simple and require little or no equipment or investment, other than your own effort. However, it may be helpful to learn the basics of a few suggested techniques through the help of a professional or at least with the guidance of someone who has been practicing them for some time.

RELAXATION FACILITATORS

Water

The movement, sound, and temperature of water seems to have a relaxing effect on most of us. Watching water, listening to waves or rain, riding on a ferryboat, or slipping into a warm bubble bath or hot tub is almost certain to take the stress away from most of us.

Warm milk and honey

Drinking warm milk and honey provides a soothing experience and relaxation, attributed to the tryptophane in the milk. This relaxing combination has often been used as a sleeping aid or for withdrawal symptoms from alcohol.

Movement

(Including: dance — running — walking — yoga — stretching — tai-chi — aikido — feldenkris, etc.)

Movement exercises can be another relaxation facilitator. Your muscles, tendons, and ligaments can lock emotional tension in. Movement will release stored energy, allowing for relaxation. Aerobic movement generates endorphins, helping relieve both anxiety and depression. Movement also helps to change your focus and thought process.

Mindless activities

Mindless activities can also provide focus and movement that serve no other purpose other than to relax. Whittling, rubbing a worry stone, and doodling are a few examples that require little or no thought, talent, or training but calm and distract us.

Music

Singing and music in general can elevate or sooth your feelings and even generate endorphins, depending on the kind of music you select. Uninhibited singing is also a way of expressing your feelings that can dispel the negative emotions and elevate the positive feelings.

Soothing sounds

Listening to birds, wind chimes, music or ocean sounds can be very calming. Even listening to another person talk can be a type of meditation, if you do it correctly. If you listen to a person's words without judgement or analysis of what they could mean, or listen without planning a response to what was said—taking in words and doing nothing with them, you will soon notice a calmness overtaking you. This method is also excellent for hearing more accurately and establishing good communications with others.

Breathing

Breathing can affect you in different ways depending on your needs. Slow, rhythmic, elongated breaths without straining are most apt to be relaxing. Entire books on breathing exercises are available. The breathing exercises can be practiced on occasion as necessary, or they may may be practiced daily for years.

Art

Art activities, such as drawing, painting, sculpting, or crafts in wood, plastics, metals, or leather are often used in psychiatric hospitals and prisons to mellow out inmates. It can be tranquilizing to work with your hands or in any creative manner that switches your focus and allows you to express your feelings without being dependent on words.

Balance skills

Juggling or balancing requires intense concentration (i.e., focus). To pause for even an instant, means loss of the harmony, and things fall apart. This is certainly not the deepest form of relaxation, but it brings an alert attention when over-stimulated senses cannot find a focus. It can also be fun and entertaining and it helps to recall the child in you—that part of you that is the creative and imaginative problem solver. Juggling may be used as a transition step into more deeply relaxing states.

Touching

(Including: massage — hugs — reflexology — acupressure — rolfing — chiropractic — naprapathy — shiatsu).

All of these are wonderful forms of communicating and breaking down strained defense barriers through touch, which the skin (the largest organ of the body) needs for positive survival. These healing procedures and/or tactile expressions are extremely relaxing and generate endorphins which help generate positive secure feelings. Even the person doing the touching will benefit by feeling more relaxed.

Sexual release

Sexual release is also a means of letting go to relax. A normal healthy body prepares to have a sexual encounter many times each day. If a person does not respond to this a few or more times each week, tension will build. Although it may not be consciously realized, it could be acted out with inappropriate eating. In the absence of a loving partner, fantasy and masturbation are normal, healthy substitutes. Because education in human sexuality is so lacking in the U.S. and being comfortable with one's own sexuality is important to a balanced, healthful life, counseling with a professional specialist in this field may be helpful, especially if fears, impotence or discomfort exist.

Imagination

(Including: Imagery — fantasy — visualizations — dreams.)

These are used for projecting what may happen and reflecting upon what did happen, giving a person the power to move emotions up or down. Mental pictures stimulate your emotions, and most people never learn to utilize them in ways that aid with stress or reaching potentials. Your vision enables creativity, motivation, dealing with fears, wish fulfillments and, ultimately, improved self-image. Learning how to direct and manage this element of yourself is a major step toward self-responsibility, self-awareness, and self-actualization. They are the key to your emotional harmony and, thus, to your very meaning/purpose in life. Books, teachers, classes, and your environment can all contribute to your learning these skills, but only practice will bring mastery.

Self-hypnosis, autogenic training, auto suggestion

These relaxation methods are very dependent upon mental pictures, along with your verbal self-direction. Using well-learned induction techniques, you guide yourself into an altered state of consciousness where you will accept suggestions that ultimately allow you to function at your best without distracting pressures. As a result, you will be doing things you could do anyway if only you did not doubt yourself. Tapes, books, classes and personal instruction from a psychologist can all result in mastery, if you will *practice, practice, practice!* If you use a tape, consider recording an induction technique using your own voice rather than that of a professional. Remember, self-efficacy is what you are seeking.

Meditation

In my opinion, meditation holds the greatest potential for deep relaxation and personal change, if it is practiced with consistency. It is always simple, available and refreshing. It can be done in many different structured forms, through physical methods such as yoga, vocal methods such as chants, or mental methods such as counting your out-breaths. Usually, visualizing is a part of the process along with a single focus. Again, remember it is the practice—not the perfection—that earns you the rewards you seek. Books, magazines, teachers, television shows, classes, and audio or video tapes are available to teach you meditation methods.

Counting

Counting down is especially good for going to sleep. Count down from 1000, visualizing each number you count. Also, with each number you count, breathe slowly, fill your lungs all the way up, and then breath out in the same manner during each count. It helps to visualize this process as you do the number you are counting. With both your mind and your body working together and occupied, stressful thoughts are unavailable, and you relax. As in all relaxation methods, it is important to be patient, not demanding, with yourself.

Biofeedback

Biofeedback is another form of meditation. It is done by attaching yourself to electronic equipment that measures a bodily function, such as brain waves, muscle tension, skin response or temperature, respiration rate, and blood pressure. The measurements can be immediately associated with the level of your stress or relaxation and will give you feedback with lights, sounds, or gauges. Americans tend to like this technique because it is quick, gives specific information, and is scientific. It can be learned simply by taking your own pulse while you watch a clock or with the aid of multi-measurement machines with lights, whistles, and printouts for $40.00 or more per session. Books and low-cost home equipment are also available to learn from.

Muscle releaxation

Progressive muscle relaxation is a simple method you can use anywhere, at anytime with no equipment. While seated or in a prone position, close your eyes and visualize your feet. Contract the muscles in your feet as tightly as you can for five seconds and then totally and suddenly relax your feet as you breathe gently. Next, focus on your calf muscles, repeating the process and isolating them from the muscles around them. It is the focus in your mind and the isolating of some muscles from the other muscles, that requires the concentration which allows you to relax. Move from one muscle group to another with this process all the way up to the top of your head, tightening, holding, isolating, focusing, and relaxing as you go, while breathing in a gentle, easy, relaxed manner. Practice, and you can't miss.

Implosive therapy

Implosive therapy invites you to bring into your mind the thoughts you have been straining to push out of your mind. Instead of distracting yourself from stressful ideas, encourage and expand on them. Using imagery, attempt to exaggerate that which upsets you to the point that it is totally unrealistic. Once you have become comfortable with the worst in your mind, reality is much easier to confront.

Paradoxical intention

Paradoxical intention works best with implosive therapy. In this case. you strain to feel what you have been avoiding. If you strain to feel angry while looking in the mirror, you will laugh. If you strain to relax, you'll be tense and visa-versa. For this method to work, you must put forth a sincere, strained effort.

Bioenergetics

Bioenergetics is the release of emotional energy stored in your physical body. Activities like screaming, yelling, hitting soft things, and physically acting out your feelings bring a release that allows for calmness. Professional assistance should be obtained when learning the whys and wherefores of these methods.

Nutrition

Nutrition from your regular meals and/or supplementation can be very important in preventing distress and encouraging relaxation. Simply eating high amounts of complex carbohydrates as recommended in the System for Healthful Eating (Chapter 7) will help you to deal with the physical and emotional aspects of stress. Staying away from refined sugars and food additives, and especially caffeine, will also contribute to an avoidance of distress symptoms. When you are under stress, it is possible to develop deficiencies of vitamins B and C, calcium or magnesium because the body uses them up more rapidly, especially if you drink alcohol, smoke, or use certain drugs. Some supplements, such as niacin, can be helpful for some people, provided they don't have high blood pressure. Also, some herb teas, such as chamomile, valerian, comfrey, or commercial blends, such as Sleepytime by Celestial Seasonings, may add to a more relaxed mood. Seeking professional advice from an herbalist, a nutritionist with a well-rounded background, or a physician who has acquired nutritional training beyond his/her medical program is also recommended.

Sensory deprivation

Sensory deprivation is a special technique not suitable for everyone. It should be employed under the supervision of a trained professional, as it could increase stress for some people. This method eliminates all stimuli. The client floats nude in a saline solution at ideal temperatures in total darkness, total silence, and total stillness for an hour or more. The effect on certain behaviors, such as smoking, can be dramatic.

Sleep

Restful sleep is restful certainly helps with the stress of physical fatigue or recovery from the stress of illness or injury. Nutrition habits, anxieties, and dreams can determine how restful your sleep is. Sleep is sometimes overused to escape a threatening world (psycho-asthenia). Drugs, smoking, and illness also can interfere with sleep patterns. It is best not to eat for two or three hours before bedtime. Current research indicates that most people do much better on at least eight hours of sleep. The time of day you sleep is important, as is the amount of light in the room. Learning a relaxation technique to put yourself to sleep can also be helpful. If you have continuing difficulties with sleep, it would beneficial to visit a sleep disorder center for specific diagnosis and corrective measures.

Smells

Smell memory is not only the strongest of our memories but it is also strongly linked to our emotions (especially from childhood). Knowing which smells effect which emotions could prove most helpful. Yale researchers learned that the smell of spiced apples can decrease stress and increase alertness, reduce blood pressure, and wake up metabolism. Check out your local lotion, spice or herb store. Know your scents and use them where you need them.

It is important to remember that we are all unique in some way, and developing our own special routines to deal with our stress is probably a good idea. As you learn any of these techniques, be patient with yourself, forgive yourself when you get off track, and do not be critical when you make a mistake or are slow to learn. Encourage yourself with positive self-talk. The relaxation method or methods that are most apt to be used well by you are the ones you believe will be helpful. The method you choose is not the concern, but how you use it and how you feel about it makes the difference.

Developing your consciousness of stress/distress and your level of confidence in dealing with it will make a difference in how many hugs you continue to seek from the refrigerator. It can also make the difference in opening or blocking your potentials for joy, good relationships, health, and general success.

When you are living a healthful lifestyle and learning to believe in yourself, you will be able to seek challenges and change, you will thrive on it instead of avoiding it! When you are relaxed, you are at your best. You have no pretenses to cover your best abilities. Your intellect is sharper, your creativity is heightened, your humor is keen, your perspective is broader, your ability to be empathetic is expanded, your usable energy is increased and not wasted spinning your wheels. And most importantly, in my opinion, when you are relaxed is the only time you can truly get outside yourself and beyond your own emotional needs in order to be able to love another person fully and not to expect anything in return.

The higher the priority you give to learning and using your ability to deal with your emotions, to being centered, balanced, calm, relaxed, tranquil, peaceful, and loving, the higher the quality of everything in all aspects of your life will be. We need our emotions, and even some useful stresses, to reach peak experiences in our lives; however, we don't need all the pitfalls that excess distress can cause. You're the boss of your life. I hope your decisions will be worthy of you.

Chapter 7

THE SYSTEM FOR
HEALTHFUL EATING

*L*ouise laughed and blushed when I first asked her if she had ever been on a weight loss diet before. She had tried *all* of the popular diets over the years, at least for a few days. Some of them, such as Weight Watchers, she had tried several times. She had tried a water fast, a liquid protein fast, the Atkins diet, the high-fiber diet—but the only time she had stayed with a reducing diet long enough to even come close to her ideal weight was when she took diet pills prescribed to her by a medical doctor.

Even during the years she was enrolled in my wellness weight loss program, Louise used several extreme diets, such as the grapefruit, rice, and the "rotation" diets. Louise had a collection of diet books larger than my own. In addition to the information Louise had gained from her extensive library, she had taken several correspondence courses in nutrition and had attended many nutrition workshops. Even though each new weight loss diet plan would come to the same end as the ones before it, Louise was still ready to optimistically embrace the next variation. It could definitely be said that Louise had a broad knowledge of nutrition, acquired from many "authorities" on the subject. Now whenever Louise thinks of going back to college, it is always to become a registered dietician.

Whenever we spoke of the unlikely possibility that any diet could change her behavior, Louise was in intellectual agreement. Emotionally, however, she would still cling to the hope that somehow the right diet combinations, timed right, with the right taste, right quantity, volume and variety would come along. When she had found this magic combination,

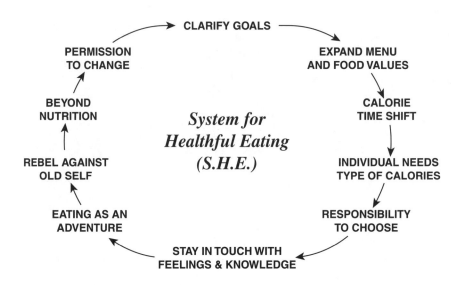

The System for Healthful Eating.

she wouldn't feel like she was on a diet, and "it" would work, and she would become thin. Midway through our work together, Louise decided that just getting the weight off would not assure her of keeping it off, so she gave up pursuing the rapid weight loss methods. Also, she decided that, in spite of some genetic heritage, her social and cultural conditioning, as well as the always-present, easy access to tempting fattening foods, it would still be possible for her to lose weight.

Having plenty of good information on healthful (and non-fattening) foods, letting go of the need for quick weight loss and all the old excuses for easy weight gain, Louise had moved herself further along the path of meaningful change to long-term success.

A Gallup survey referenced in the March 1990 issue of *American Health* offered clear indications that like Louise, many Americans are making some positive changes when it comes to food. Crash diet programs are losing much of their old appeal. Getting rid of fat, junk foods, and protein fasting powders in favor of fruits and vegetables seems to be the new direction. Only three percent of the people surveyed found that special diet foods were helpful in losing weight, and only one percent credited diet books. As a society, we are finally becoming aware that complex carbohydrates not only do not cause weight gain, but actually help us a great deal, especially if we exercise in a reasonable manner. Meanwhile, it appears that we are still emotional eaters, as we seem to crave the comfort of chocolate and ice cream while at the same time we want to lose weight.

Unlike Louise, many people do not have all the latest information regarding nutrition and weight loss. New, relevant information is bombarding us at such a rapid pace that is difficult for even specialists in the field to keep up with the data—not to mention the average person.

Studies of eating patterns and weight, such as those by Dr. Colin Campbell of Cornell University, have been going on for years. His study, which took place in China, is so vast and the numbers so mind boggling, that it has only recently begun to hit the popular press, and it will take a good deal longer for it to become familiar to the general population. One of Dr.Campbell's many interesting findings is that, while eating substantially more calories than the average overweight American, Chinese people in certain geographic areas do not develop weight problems. These people eat a low fat, high carbohydrate diet from local foods that are not processed or packaged. This finding indicates that it is not the *volume* of calories, but the *type* of calories that makes the difference where weight problems are concerned. The China study is discussed in more detail later in this chapter.

Dr. William H. Lee, in *Health News & Review*, January/February 1987, lets us know that the more you diet, the greater the percentage of food that ends up in the fat cells. This can mean that after the initial weight loss that results from most reducing diets, you can actually gain weight while eating less. The body produces more enzymes which are used to store fat. And, of course, people in the public eye, for example Oprah Winfrey, have allowed us to see and hear that quick weight loss through fasting is certainly not the resolution to weight problems. In fact, on her show which aired in Arizona on November 5, 1990, Oprah, having regained the weight she had recently lost on a fasting program, declared that she would never go on another diet and certainly would never fast again.

Even though the bulk of the information and the basic message contained in my book, *Change Your Mind: Change Your Weight* (Health

Plus Publishers, 1985) is still valid today, if I were writing the book now, I would make some changes, including the elimination of nine pages devoted to types of weight loss diets. Although the breakdown of how the different diets work might be interesting, it has little to do with long-term success, other than to distract individuals from it and postpone it, possibly causing some psychological damage in the process.

We now know that all weight loss diets are the wrong approach to weight loss, and to focus on them, even as a temporary solution, is counterproductive. Any very-low-calorie diet is apt to end up causing problems rather than providing solutions—and some of the problems are potentially fatal.

In 1985, along with giving information on weight loss diets, I was also saying such things as, "a person who has learned to listen to his or her own body has become sensitive to hearing the subtle, and sometimes not so subtle, messages it gives." When these natural sensitivity skills are combined with some basic knowledge of nutrition and a commitment to label reading, weight loss diets, as such, are seen as a frivolous waste of time, energy, money, and health. I also stated that "when you are in the bookstore looking for a diet book, remember—it's not the quantity of weight you lose that's so important, it's the quality of the weight you lose and your attitudes about it. You want to find a weight loss program that (1) does not put you in medical jeopardy; (2) that encourages weight loss mainly from fat stores, not from muscle mass or through dehydration; and (3) aids you in developing a greater belief in your own ability to determine your eating habits and weight."

Now, in 2000, I believe the only weight loss program that really has an excellent chance of working is a program developed by the individual who is going to use it. In addition, the program should be focused on health. It should be comprehensive in scope, done without fanfare or special products, and allow changes to come about slowly as the individual learns to prefer new healthful tastes and builds a diet for life. In this chapter, I have put those ideas into a system from which you can build your eating program. I know if you try to control your eating behavior through a plan structured by someone else, you will eventually rebel. Worse, you won't be building the much-needed confidence in yourself to be able to take charge of yourself and your own eating habits.

Since 1985, I have come to be even more sure about my belief in a vegetarian diet, and that the closer you come to eating a vegan (no animal products) vegetarian diet, the healthier you will be and the less likely to encounter weight problems. I have yet to see a longtime vegan vegetarian who is overweight. I am not saying it isn't possible, because we know that a vegan could eat large amounts of refined sugars, salt, high-fat nuts, seeds, and fruits such as avocados. This is, however, unlikely, since the person who has been interested enough to have been a vegan for some time is also going to be very interested in health and will go out of his or her way to avoid potentially harmful or fattening foods. In May of 1991, Dr. Richard Adamson, the Director of Etiology for the National Cancer Institute, was quoted as stating research in the U.S. and Japan confirms his own findings that carcinogen compounds are formed in cooked meat and fish. They are formed by heating of any animal protein—they can not be avoided simply by eliminating some meats. This means that all animal products are unsafe, even in small amounts. Current research corroborates these claims.

I have been a vegetarian since 1976, with all the benefits and inconveniences that entails, and I know I have come to prefer it over all other ways of eating. But, as I've often said to Louise, I don't recommend that anyone suddenly and dramatically take up this lifestyle as they are likely to burn out on it quickly. I also know that an overweight person can become trim without becoming a vegetarian. To me, however, it is the best way for the overweight person to gradually become healthy and slim.

Louise found the idea of becoming a vegan vegetarian somewhat overwhelming, but she has also come to realize that extreme weight loss diets such as those she had tried in the past are also very hard to live with. Now, she has accepted the idea of building her own diet over a long period of time, and it is coming more easily. She has taken many of her old recipes for fattening foods and modified them by substituting healthful ingredients. She does not have to grapple with issues of control or dependency and the changes are gradual. In her path to change, she is learning to relax and find harmony between the emotions she creates in her mind and her knowledge and sense of her own body and what it needs.

Louise's struggle within herself, and her struggles with the weight loss authorities have ended, so she has only her own impatience to deal with. If you see the following food choice system, which I call the System for Healthful Eating (S.H.E.), as a resource from which to build your own diet, although it may take some time and seem difficult now and then, you will be much more willing to accept your own changes and give yourself the credit you deserve.

Other resources for building healthful diets are all around you. The trick is to seek them out as you need them. Specialists in the field love to be asked questions, but *you* have the responsibility to ask them for what you do with the information.

THE SYSTEM FOR HEALTHFUL EATING

The System for Healthful Eating (S.H.E.) will allow you to achieve personalized, healthful eating preferences.

Weight loss diets have contributed far more to fat gains than to long-term fat losses for millions of people struggling to master their corpulence. Counting calories has proven to be aversive, and structured weight loss diets deny individual free choices (a sense of taking charge of yourself). They also do not allow for hour-to-hour, day-to-day changes in one's nutritional needs. If you are ever going to prefer healthful foods, enjoy their tastes, expand the variety of foods you eat, and have ample volume to satisfy your hunger, changes will have to come not only from your environment, but also from within you.

Changes in your attitudes (i.e., "I can never like green stuff"), value priorities (i.e., I always stay up to watch late-night TV and I'm too tired to get up early enough to exercise before going to work), and your perception of your ability to eat in your own best interest (i.e., "I'll always prefer a good steak to a salad, and I'll always need some help to control my eating!") are essential. Highly structured weight loss diets are infantilizing and demeaning, and they take away from your reasons to believe in yourself.

Worse, weight loss diets set up a control/dependency factor against which to rebel (i.e., "I was bad yesterday—I cheated on my diet, ha-ha!"). Weight loss diets imply that you are somehow inadequate and that you are not intelligent enough to make logical choices on your own. The goal is for you to be able, with confidence, to make informed, independent, spontaneous decisions about what you eat each, knowing the food will fill you, satisfy you, meet your nutritional needs, and be enjoyable to your taste. You do not need mighty stores of will power to force and control yourself in a struggle that will only exhaust and defeat you in the end. Nor do you need a Ph.D. in nutrition. Simply lead the way through the following steps of your choice with the courage and sense of adventure you've always had, but may have been afraid or reluctant to take advantage of.

1. *Clarify your goals.*

Changing the volume, quality, and frequency of what you eat are ultimately important, but not nearly as important as changing your beliefs about your ability to change to healthful food preferences, and handling the feelings that drive you to the cupboard. These changes are far more valuable than quick, temporary weight loss. People who make sudden, radical changes in their diets will burn out quickly and regain a higher percentage of body fat than they had to start with. If you feel that you must force your self-control, pushing your logical will against your emotional desires, it is then only a matter of time until your defenses become fatigued and your emotions take over. A sincere commitment to change, the image you have of yourself, the quality of your life, and how you are motivated is far more important to achieving long-term weight loss and satisfaction with the lifestyle that keeps the weight off.

As an improvement over weight-loss diets, S.H.E. is intended to serve as a guide to your own individual efforts to gradually expand your food choices and preferences. A 1990 study by Dr. Judith S. Stern, Professor of nutrition and internal medicine at the University of California at Davis, found that the dieters most likely to keep the extra pounds they had lost off were those who had designed their own programs. Modify your old menu by replacing or eliminating most of the fat and refined sweeteners and flours. The following are steps in a process of learning to *prefer* healthful, high performance, mood-enhancing additions to your usual menu. Remind yourself frequently of your goals.

2. *Expand your menu choices and decide on food values.*

Additions to your menu are most apt to become taste preferences when you add new foods gradually (1-2 new food items at a time) and become psychologically comfortable with these additions before introducing additional new food items. When you learn to prefer foods that help you, the mental struggle between what your emotions tell you that you want and what your logic tells you that you should eat is over. When you are at the grocery store, the cafe, or looking into your refrigerator and not using a structured diet, consider the following important factors in making decisions about what you want to achieve in your eating habits.

- When you consider eating a new food (or any food), examine it and determine what is in it and what value it may have to you. If you are uncertain of the contents or how it may affect your nutritional interests, hold off on buying it or eating it until you can determine how useful it may be to you. It may be helpful to carry a small pocket book containing information on the nutritional value of foods until such time as you can make most of your decisions with ease.

- When considering a new food or recipe, it is psychologically important to open your mind and free yourself of prejudgments and predeterminations. Remind yourself that you are adaptable! Your goal is to improve your belief in your ability to adjust your taste preferences to your physical and mental needs. Your self-talk and mental images can serve you in this effort. Telling yourself you won't like a new food or can't stand a food that will serve you well is a sure way to keep the old preferences. Likewise, trying to convince yourself you love something new can also backfire. If you will allow for a neutral position by deciding you will repeatedly eat a new food for a 6-10 week period before you make a judgement as to whether or not you like it, you will give yourself time to accept it. Once you have accepted the food, continued use will lead to appreciation, and gradually appreciation will become preference, as long as you are not talking yourself out of it. You have already come to like foods you once didn't. Use those memories to aid you. Let down your defenses—permit change.

3. *Gradually shift evening calories to morning hours.*

The time of day you eat is extremely important. The volume and type of calories that can lead to weight gain in the afternoon or evening can actually help you achieve weight loss if you eat them during the morning hours. Your body needs more fuel and assimilates and burns foods better in the morning, while its efficiency wanes as the day wears on, until you reach the danger zone of 7:00 p.m. to bedtime. Eating a larger balanced breakfast and lunch is best achieved gradually, as is the gradual introduction of new food options. As you add to your morning meal, you are able to gradually alter your evening meal and the type of calories you consume at that time. Mental fatigue or tension at the end of the day adds to your appetite, so exercise or even a casual walk to relieve these will reduce food drives.

4. *Choose the type of calories that meet your needs.*

"Maintaining weight loss is the antithesis of counting every calorie," says Dr. Judith Rodin, Chair of psychology at Yale University, as quoted by *American Health Magazine*, Spring, 1991. *All calories are not the same.* Protein and complex carbohydrates burn 2-1/2 times faster than fat. Complex carbohydrates are very difficult for your body to store as fat. They are stored as glycogen in the muscles and liver to provide energy which is quickly used. Also, one gram of fat has nine calories, compared with four calories per gram of carbohydrate or protein. Protein must be broken down and reassembled before it can be stored, and this process burns calories. However, carefully consider your sources of protein. If you acquire your protein mostly from animal products, you will also get a great many unwanted fat calories, not to mention a lot of chemicals you don't need. The small amount of protein that you do need (5 percent of your total calories) can be obtained from plant sources at a much lower cost in fat. Grains such as amaranth (a complete protein), beans such as defatted soy, pinto, and garbanzo, along with a few nuts, seeds and sprouts, will serve you well as sources of protein. Refined carbohydrates (sugars/flours) are empty calories you can do without, as they too are easily stored as fat. A true vegetarian diet implies a variety of plant foods are consumed, and these will supply the eight essential amino acids, and more. Some individuals follow "junk food diets" which, while they do not include meant, cannot be considered true vegetarian diets.

5. *Follow these guidelines for healthful food choices.*

Choose your foods for more than their tastes and the fact that they momentarily satisfy your emotional needs. Choose foods for lifelong healthful weight. In April 1991, Neal Barnard, M.D., of the Physicians Committee for Responsible Medicine, proposed new basic four food groups to prevent heart disease, stroke, diabetes, and cancer. The proposed groups consist of: 1) grains, 2) fruits, 3) vegetables, 4) legumes; and no animal products. If you learn only the following guide from which to select your foods, you have enough information to make wise choices. Simply keep a balance of the items marked with one asterisk (*) and two asterisks (**) from the various food categories. And, stay with quantities in correct ratio to your body's needs, especially during the evening meal.

CRITERIA FOR HEALTHFUL FOOD SELECTIONS

The foods listed below are divided into six major categories. Within the categories, food items are marked with either one, two, or three asterisks (*, **, or ***). Those that are marked with * are recommended for health and weight loss. These foods and beverages include fresh foods, free of pesticides when possible (although frozen foods may actually be fresher than fresh foods depending on storage and freezing methods; food with high nutritional values and high fiber rather than calories from fat; pure water (for drinking and cooking).

Foods marked with ** contain little or no refined carbohydrates, little or no refined sugars or flours, and little or no added salt or chemicals. These foods can be used in moderation, but make sure to monitor fat and toxin content.

Foods marked with *** contain animal fat, and are not recommended in a healthful diet; you may want to include them in the beginning, gradually eliminating them from your diet as healthful options increase.

In April 1991, in the *New England Journal of Medicine*, Dr. Walter Willett and Dr. Frank M. Sacks of Harvard University reported on their research relating food to cancer and other illness. They stated, "The optimal intake of cholesterol is probably zero," "meaning the avoidance of all animal products," adding, "avoid all fats from land mammals—especially lard, red meat, and dairy products."

Mixing * foods from the various categories will provide the ultimate in healthful diets. Foods marked with ** can be included in moderation, and foods with *** should gradually be eliminated from your diet as you learn to prefer more healthful food choices.

A. COMPLEX CARBOHYDRATES

Should account for approximately 70 to 80 percent of diet

*   Wide variety of vegetables (especially greens)

*   Whole fruits

*   Variety of 100% whole grains

*   Variety of legumes (i.e., peas and beans)

**   Seeds and nuts

B. PROTEINS

The World Health Organization recommends 5 to 10 percent of diet be comprised of protein

*   Defatted soy products (tofu, tempeh, soy isolate)

*   Beans, peas, lentils

*   100% whole grains (particularly amaranth and quinoa)

*   Sprouts (vegetables, grains, beans, etc.)

**   Seeds and nuts (almonds, sesame)

**   Fresh fish (not shell fish)

**   Skim milk dairy products (if not allergic)

*** Cheese (high in fat and salt)

*** Meats (contain a high percentage of fat and cholesterol) Meats are stored most easily as fat; usually contains chemical preservatives, growth hormones, antibiotics nitrates and nitrites. The average American diet consists of 40 percent protein, mostly from animal products. Meat has high association with major illnesses, causes calcium loss and other medical problems, such as certain cancers and cardiovascular problems. Meat has no fiber.

C. FATS & OILS

  * Fruits (avocados)

  ** Cooking oils (Prefer mono-unsaturated, such as extra virgin, cold-pressed olive oil stored in a dark bottle. Keep cool. Avoid saturated and poly-unsaturated oils.)

  ** Nuts & seeds (almonds, sesame)

  ** Grains (corn)

  *** Animal products - high in saturated fats

D. FIBER

  * Fruits (figs)

  * Grains (oats)

  * Vegetables (cabbage)

  ** Nuts (almonds)

E. SWEETENERS

  * Whole fruits

  ** Fruit juice

  ** Honey and maple syrup (even in their natural form, these are high in calories and are easily stored as fat)

  *** Refined sugars from grains, beets, cane, and fruit

  *** Artificial sweeteners (Nutrasweet)

G. LIQUIDS

  * Water (pure, clean)

*   Vegetable juices

*   Herb teas (caffeine free)

*   Broth (fat free, beware of sodium)

**   Fruit juices

**   Beer (grain beverage, alcohol free)

Here's a few things to keep in mind when planning your healthful eating system:

- Grocery shopping is "safer" when you aren't stressed, fatigued, or hungry.

- Going grocery shopping once each week offers less exposure to temptation.

- Lean cupboards keep tough decisions to a minimum.

- Fattening foods, such as nuts, are better purchased in small amounts.

- When eating with friends, make your preferences known in advance. You can learn to say "no" in a non-offensive way.

- You will find that many restaurants will try to meet your needs if you give them the chance.

No one else will ever be able to monitor your nutritional needs better than you. It is up to each of us to become sensitive to our body's needs and knowledgeable about food values. Also, if you are ever to gain the confidence you want, it must come through your own insights and efforts. Therefore, it is important that you make the food choices necessary to your own well-being and not just follow some authority's directives. If you need information, use professionals as resources, not as parental figures to be dependent on. Step 5 is another resource to consult. *You* determine the choices and take responsibility to apply the information to your needs.

6. *Stay in touch with your feelings and learn what your nutritional need are.*

Understanding and sensing your nutritional needs leads to an ability to make spontaneous choices that work for you in each new situation. An understanding comes from collecting basic information and learning how to apply it to specific needs (i.e., you need carbohydrates to jog a 10K). It is not necessary to become a nutritionist; however, asking questions of one, reading a book or two on the subject, or taking a class can get you started. Once you have some general information, you can stay on top of new information by reading. Nutritional newsletters, monthly health magazines (such as *Vegetarian Times* and *American Health*), and even the daily newspaper are good sources of current information. If you read what five different nutritionists have to say, you will find some differences as well as some similarities. This can seem confusing, but remember, it is your own unique body that really tells the story. Take into consideration all that you have become aware of from the nutritionists, especially when you find most of them in agreement.

But even more important is listening to what your body tells you. Within twenty minutes to a half hour after you eat, your body will tell you how well it liked what you gave it. If you are becoming tense, tired, full of gas, etc., you know something disagreed with you. If your pulse is racing, you may be having an allergic reaction. The point is that nobody can know better than you how your food is affecting you if you learn to sense and listen to what your body is telling you.

7. *Think of eating as an adventure.*

Discovering how food works is much more exciting than the denial, forcing, controlling and calorie-counting that goes with typical weight-loss diets. Your body's needs are constantly changing with age and levels of stress, pollution, physical activities, etc. Hour-to-hour, day-to-day and year-to-year, your physical, emotional, and mental needs continually change. Your adventure, then, becomes the search for the foods that will fuel your needs as they arise; always seeking maximal performance, optimal energy levels, calmness, and health. Using food to provide entertainment, companionship, emotional comforting, social rewards and sexual gratification, or to fulfill other non-nutritional needs, leaves much to be desired. The joy and the sensual satisfaction of eating can be enhanced as you expand your choices that have value to you, with no cause for feeling guilty.

8. *Rebel against your old self.*

S.H.E. represents your choices that can help you create a more positive self-image. S.H.E. is not your controlling parents, spouse, boss, doctor, or the dietician upon whom you may feel dependent. If you feel the need to rebel against something, let it be your old ways of thinking and behaving. You may not want to even be aware of such struggles going on because it may not seem to make sense to you. If you join a weight loss program because you feel too weak to help yourself, you are apt to come to both praise and resent that program, and consciously or subconsciously you may rebel against it. Most of us don't want to be controlled. Perfectionists seek out structure, which feels like control, because they don't trust themselves to perform well without a lot of exacting guidelines, so they can be sure to tell if they will get a gold star for their performance (please others). If they start out doing well, then it is because of the program, and they are dependent on the program. Then they begin to resent the program upon which they've become dependent because their dependency points out a weakness in themselves. They become angry and fearful and they rebel against the dependency and the controller (i.e., the program). To avoid this, drop your defenses, and allow yourself to see this is your self-made program. Remember that S.H.E. is only a resource in your effort to take charge of your life.

9. *Think beyond nutrition.*

Supportive activities in developing healthful eating:

- Clarify your philosophy of life
- Clarify your value priorities
- Base your decisions on your values and beliefs
- Practice listening to your feelings, even when they are mild
- Monitor your self-talk and use affirmations
- Monitor your mental images—give yourself non-food rewards for self-enhancing behavior
- Practice relaxation techniques (e.g., meditation)
- During stressful times, keep a broad perspective of your life

- Confront your fears (desensitize yourself to them)

- Keep expectations moderate

- Clarify your strongest motivations and use them to change yourself

- Nurture your ability to love in loving relationships

- Develop open and honest communication skills

- Practice listening without judgement, analysis, or preparing a response.

- Do aerobic exercise for a minimum of four times each week for 30 minutes; and/or 60 seconds (e.g., jog in place) for those moments when you are apt to eat inappropriately due to emotional hunger.

- Store only those foods you need for the coming week

- Use your support system when you feel overwhelmed taking the risks of changing

- Have a regular sexual release (3 or more times per week)

- Read some resources offering nutritional information weekly

- Bring your lunch if healthful alternatives aren't available.

10. *Give yourself permission to change.*

Allowing change in yourself works much better than forcing or controlling change. Forcing and controlling exhausts you and encourages your desire to stay with the old ways. To be in harmony of body and mind, thus achieving a relaxed balance of logic and emotion, let go of:

- Ego struggles and internal conflicts of right and wrong

- Avoiding your fears—instead, move toward fears on your own terms

- Forcing yourself to eat inappropriately (i.e., diets).

THE CHINA DIET STUDY

Prior to beginning to make your own healthful food choices from the food groups listed in Step 5, you may wish to consider some of the findings from the unprecedented nutritional study carried out by Dr. T. Colin Campbell of Cornell University, often referred to as the China Diet Dtudy.

Obesity is related more to *what* people eat than how much they eat. "We're basically a vegetarian species and should be eating a wide variety of plant foods and minimizing our intake of animal products," said Dr. Campbell in an interview with Jane Brody published in *The New York Times*. Dr. Campbell was the key U.S. figure in a cooperative epidemiological study with the Chinese, British, and Americans. This study looked at 367 factors in 6,500 Chinese subjects, dealing with lifestyle, nutritional intake, health status, and mortality since 1983. It is the biggest study of its kind ever undertaken and the results will be years in completion. The preliminary findings clearly point to the fact that the more animal fat we consume, the greater our chances of premature death from cancer, heart disease, and other major killers (see references cited at end of this chapter).

Allowing for height adjustment, the Chinese consume 20 percent more calories than Americans do, but Americans are 25 percent fatter. Americans eat more fat; Chinese eat more starch. The Chinese eat only one-third of the fat of the average American, while eating twice the starch. The data concerning the role of exercise is not yet in.

In making your food choices, you might want to consider that the current recommendations of the American Dieticians Association, which suggest a maximum of 30 percent of calories from fat, may still be too high to adequately lower the risk of heart disease and cancer. The China Study suggests a maximum of 20 percent of total calories from fat, but realistically only 10 to 15 percent or less should be eaten to minimize health risks.

A diet high in animal protein is linked to chronic disease. Americans eat a third more protein than the Chinese, and 70 percent of it comes from animal products, compared with 7 percent animal protein for the Chinese. A high protein diet may promote rapid growth in early life, but it increases the risk of cancer in later life.

Most Chinese consume no dairy products, obtaining most of their calcium from vegetables. Although they consume only half the calcium Americans do, osteoporosis is very uncommon in China. This is likely to be because greater animal protein intake is associated with increased calcium needs. Dairy calcium intake does not reduce the risk of osteoporosis; in fact, it may very likely increase it. Vegetarians tend to have lower calcium needs and a lower risk of osteoporosis. High sodium intake also increases the need for calcium.

The range of blood cholesterol values in the U.S. population is said to be 155 to 274 mg/dl. Almost all the China group values are between 88 to 165 mg./dl. Most importantly, "coronary heart disease risk in the China study continues to decline to an almost negligible level when cholesterol levels are low." Colon cancer risk correlates in exactly the same way. The same is true for animal protein, which is 0 to 20 percent for the China group and 70 percent for the Americans. The study found less of a risk for disease in those who eat the least amount of animal protein.

Dr. Campbell stated, "a diet that minimizes the intake of animal food might optimize reduction of the risk of both communicable and degenerative diseases at the same time." It is becoming increasingly clear that a vegetarian approach to eating offers the least risk for these diseases. For more information on the China Diet Study, refer to the references cited at the end of this chapter.

THREE-PHASE TRANSITIONAL MENU

The three-phase gradual transition menu found at the end of this chapter provides only an example of how to eat healthy. It is not a recipe book. In fact, the recipes with which you are most apt to stick with are the ones you create yourself by modifying the ingredients of your old recipes to create healthful, non-fattening foods. The idea is to proceed slowly with your menu alterations and to own your changes. Proceeding slowly and owning your changes statistically offers the best chance for success over the long term.

Eventually, the goal is to move from an inappropriate way of eating to a more healthful approach. If your changes are gradual and you do not mentally resist or push yourself, they will become your preferred choices as well.

Each phase we have supplied in this sample menu adds twelve new alternatives to the old cycle of food choices. The important factors being considered in this three phase progression are: fats, refined flours and sweeteners, salt, fiber, protein, and carbohydrates. The intent is to gradually reduce total fats, especially saturated fat. Mono-unsaturated or polyunsaturated oils are preferred.

The same idea is also true of refined cereals or flours. Whole grains are preferred whenever possible. Sweeteners are to be gradually reduced to a more subtle taste, using whole fruits as the sweetener preferred over artificial and refined sweeteners. All forms of salt are also gradually reduced and eliminated whenever possible. Protein is intended to be reduced far below that of the standard American diet. As mentioned, the World Health Organization indicates that the necessary protein needs comprise no more than 5 to 10 percent of the total adult diet. Pregnant and lactating women and growing children require 2 percent more.

Each phase includes increases in fiber and the percentage of complex carbohydrates. Simple carbohydrates are decreased in each phase by reducing old choices. In the end, total carbohydrate intake will ideally be 70 to 80 percent of the total diet.

In phase I, gradually add new menu items, such as the examples given or others from the cookbooks and resources referred to in Appendix A. Do this progressively through each of the three phases over a period of three to six months' time, so that twelve new menu items for each meal will be available and will gradually come to dominate the overall menu. What is eaten most often comes to be preferred, if it is not mentally resisted. Focus on how the food can serve your desired goals.

Choose from the twelve more menu items and/or recipes for each of the daily meals: breakfast, lunch, and dinner. As indicated earlier, these are to be interchanged with your own usual menu items more and more frequently as you move through each phase. The menu items given in Phase I may be used in Phase II, and Phase II items can be used in Phase III as part of moving gradually into healthful eating.

Open up to new food choices by simply accepting them with greater regularity, keeping your self-talk as neutral as possible. Your taste buds will do the changing if your old biases are out of your mind. It is not necessary to talk yourself into or out of these changes. Just permit them, and practice them. You may want to spend one to two months in each phase before moving ahead. Progress as resistance ends.

GRADUAL TRANSITIONS: A MENU FOR HEALTHFUL EATING

Weight loss diets are often unrealistic, boring, controlling and bring about burnout quickly. Partial fasting is denial and creates longings to consume fattening foods in the future. Partial fasting can also be dangerous to your health. Eating a well-balanced and healthful diet can be assimilated easily into your life, and eventually the new foods will come to be preferred by taste. To avoid feeling cheated, make sure you have a variety of healthful food choices available. If you tell yourself you will always love fattening food and you have to struggle to "control" your drive to get it, you set yourself up to avoid change.

Learning to prefer (by taste) healthful food choices is most likely to be successful over an extended period of time if you introduce the changes *gradually* and if each individual *owns* his or her changes. Personal healthful changes made in your own unique manner are more apt to work than those imposed by outside directives.

Keeping with this philosophy, the following three-phase menu should not be viewed as a diet but as an example of how you may progressively choose a more healthful way to eat that is preferred by taste and enjoyable to live with. No matter how you go about making your gradual changes, remember that you are in charge and can continue to improve your choices as your needs and life evolve. The important idea is that healthful eating becomes your personal adventure, and with it, self-awareness, growth, and ownership.

The transitional menu means that healthful food choices are mixed more and more frequently with your old menu; healthful recipes gradually dominate your menu and become the preferred choices. Even your old, fattening menu can be changed to healthful choices simply by adjusting the recipe content. Pizza, for example, can be made with a whole grain crust held together by using apple sauce and topped with "no-fat" soy cheese and vegetables and fruits instead of meat.

Eat each reconstructed recipe routinely (without judgement or expectation) until you have psychologically come to accept it. The more you eat the new ingredients, the more your taste buds will appreciate them. Gradually keep adding new choices to your menu until what is healthful far exceeds what is unhealthful, and you prefer what is healthful by taste as well as logic. Remember, the idea of telling yourself you "cannot" have old, fattening choices will make them more and more appealing to you.

During your evolving changes in learning to prefer healthful food choices, what you do (or do not do) mentally can help to ensure your success. The more neutral your self-talk remains, the less you will resist change or put pressure on yourself to make changes. Your taste preferences will change on their own when you routinely eat and mentally accept your adventure as the new you.

If you apply the knowledge you have learned in earlier chapters, your consumption of fats, refined flours, sweeteners, salt, and excess protein will decrease while your consumption of fiber and complex carbohydrates will increase.

There is no set amount of time you will remain in each phase, as long as the transitions are gradual enough for you to modify your emotional and taste preferences without resistance. When you realize changes have taken place and feel your sense of ownership/empowerment, I encourage you to enjoy it briefly, then refocus to achieve the next steps until the process brings the self-efficacy (inner magic) you will know you have earned.

As in the chapter on healthful exercise, two excellent brand names are used in the following menu. These are products I have been using for years with great satisfaction. The companies that package these products stress quality nutrition and ease of preparation which will aid you in the achievement of your goals without robbing you of your ownership of long-term success.

The following menu is not meant to be "your" menu, but only to give you an awareness of the kind of menus you can create for yourself. Ownership works!

It is common to have a menu that includes 12 to 15 items eaten routinely in a cyclical manner. You may want to define the menu that has contributed to unwanted pounds. The following are a few examples of "additions" you may make to your old menu.

Phase I

Breakfast 1
Scrambled egg substitutes & chives
100% whole grain toast with unsweetened applesauce
Fresh fruit
Herb tea

Breakfast 2
100% whole grain french toast made
with egg substitutes & almond extract
Fresh fruit & maple syrup
Herb tea

Lunch 1
Sweet potato-banana salad
100% whole grain cinnamon/raisin bagel
Fresh fruit
Non-fat frozen yogurt
Mineral water

Lunch 2
Boca Burger
100% whole grain bun
Mixed vegetable salad
Fresh fruit
Ice tea (black or green)

Dinner 1

100% whole grain spaghetti
Low fat spaghetti sauce with ground Boca Burger
Whole grain garlic bread with fat free margarine
Large vegetable salad with banana walnut dressing
Alcohol free beer

Dinner 2

Spanish brown rice with ground Boca Burger
Green beans
Mixed vegetable salad with banana almond dressing
Fresh fruit & non-dairy frozen strawberry Rice Dream
Ice water or green tea

Phase II

Breakfast 1

Kashi Cold Cereals
Fresh fruit and vanilla soy milk
Herb tea

Breakfast 2

Kashi Breakfast Pilaf
Soy milk or fruit juice
Herb tea

Lunch 1

Kashi GOLean Plus Woman - chocolate shake
Whole grain raisin muffin
Fresh vegetable plate
Herb tea

Lunch2

Fresh ten vegetable salad
Multi- whole grain blueberry bagel
Fresh fruit
Ice herb tea

Dinner 1

Whole wheat angel hair pasta
Low fat tomato sauce with Boca Burger Bits
Fresh salad and fruit
100% whole grain bread sticks
Alcohol free beer

Dinner 2

Vegetable stew with Boca Burger Bits
100% whole grain rye bread
Garden salad
Fresh fruit
Iced lemon/lime mineral water or herb tea

Phase III

Breakfast 1

Kashi Pillows with low fat soy milk
100% multi-grain toast and unsweetened preserves
Fresh fruit
Herb tea

Breakfast 2

Kashi Go and Fruit
100% Multi-grain toast with apple sauce
Fruit juice and herb tea

Lunch 1

Vegetarian chili with ground Boca Burger
Rice cakes with pureed fresh fruit
Poached pears
Flavored mineral water with ice

Lunch 2

Stuffed peppers with ground Boca Burger
100% whole grain onion bagels with hummus
Fresh fruit

Non-dairy frozen dessert
Flavored mineral water or herb tea

Dinner 1

Sweet-sour vegetable sauté
100% whole grain pita bread
Vegetable salad
Fresh fruit
Herb tea

Dinner 2

Potato casserole
100% whole grain bread
Steamed spinach
Vegetable salad
Fresh fruit
Herb tea or mineral water with ice

CHINA STUDY REFERENCES

Campbell TC: "Association of Diet and Disease: A Comprehensive Study of Health Characteristics in China. Conference on Social Consequences of Chinese Economic Reform," *Harvard University Fairbank Center on East Asian Studies*, Cambridge, MA, May 23-24, 1997.

Campbell TC, J Chen: "Diet and Health Characteristics in Rural China: Lessons Learned and Unlearned." *Nutrition Today*, 1999; 34:116-123.

Campbell TC: Critique of Report on "Food, Nutrition, and Prevention of Cancer, a Global Perspective." *Nutrition Today*, at print.

Campbell TC, J Chen: "Energy Balance: Interpretation of Data from Rural China." *Toxicol Sci*, Dec 1999; 52(2 Suppl): 87-94.

Chapter 8

HEALTHFUL EXERCISE

Losing It Your Way

While growing up, Louise was shy and non-assertive. Unless the teacher organized the playground games and required her to take part, Louise would retreat with a friend or keep to herself. She worked from junior high school on, so she never took part in the usual extra-curricular activities. Although she did have a bike, it was more for utilitarian purposes than for fun. Exercise was never something Louise enjoyed or at which she excelled. So, is it surprising that as an adult she viewed it more like the physical work she did at home or on the job? Certainly exercise wasn't something she looked forward to or to which she wanted to devote her free time. This attitude was especially true when she became a postal worker where she spent most of her working day standing on her feet.

The more Louise learned about weight problems and the heavier she grew, the more she would try to force herself into a regular routine. In the various diets and programs she would join, her efforts would be short term and often too rigorous. She would join fitness spas and aerobic dance classes, but it would be just a matter of time until the class conflicted with other, higher priorities, or her friend wasn't able to make it, or something would interfere. Louise would then be disappointed in herself and put herself down for not being able to follow through with her commitment.

After years of struggle with diet and exercise, Louise began to value exercise in a new way. Even when she was consistent for less than a few weeks, she knew her mood, energy level, attitudes, and hopefulness were

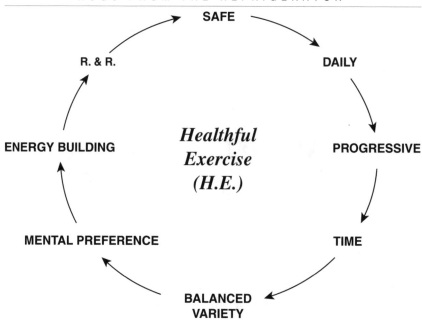

Healthful Exercise.

noticeably improved. Her weight loss efforts were clearly enhanced, her confidence level would rise, and she found herself less often in the snacking clutches of restaurants, cafés or bars for entertainment. She knew how much more satisfying it was to identify with people who value their health. Also, having read many articles and books, listened to testimonials and lectures, and counseled with exercise physiologists and weight loss specialists, it was hard for her to believe anything other than that exercise was a worthwhile activity. She was motivated and had given it a higher priority in her life. She even purchased a treadmill so that she would have no excuses about convenience or time, or appropriate clothing.

Louise injured her back at work while lifting a mail sack because her back had not been strengthened properly with healthful exercise. That is not to say that people that who are in good physical shape can't be injured, too, but usually injury happens less frequently, and when it does happen, the injury is less serious and recovery is more rapid.

After great medical expense, one operation, months of therapy, and pain that may never be completely gone, Louise is doing her exercises far more faithfully than ever before. Today she is happy just to be able to exercise at all. She is still deriving most of the benefits exercise provides and will probably continue to exercise as long as she is able—certainly not by forcing herself, which is not the recommended way to come to a point where exercise is preferred over being sedentary.

When we realize, through experience, that body movement is the only way our metabolism will be changed, or if you believe in the set point theory (i.e., that our bodies always return to the weight we are programmed to be), then the only way the set point can be changed as well as one of the ways in which we can find harmony in ourselves—we love it.

In studies from 1990, Dr. Judith S. Sterns of the University of California at Davis found the most important factor in permanent weight adjustment is physical exercise. Ninety percent of the people in the successful weight loss group used regular exercise to keep the extra weight off. If I emotionally *want* to exercise, as opposed to simply thinking I *should* exercise, and I truly believe I value exercise as a practical, important, and necessary part of my life and how I relate to others, there will be no question of whether I will exercise. The only questions will be how to fit it into my schedule consistently, and what the best ways for me to do it are.

Getting started has everything to do with staying with it. Goals are more mental than they are physical. As with diet and weight loss, you are starting out to change the way you look at yourself, including your beliefs, attitudes and priorities, and not just your behavior or body shape. You are setting out to learn to *prefer* a new aspect to your life—to get beyond struggles with yourself ("will I or won't I exercise today?"). In every sense of the word, you are intending to get married to a behavior for life. You are wanting to become sensitive to your body and everything it can teach you. You want to learn how you and your body can nurture each other; you want to love, honor, cherish, and protect one another; through a lot *less* sickness and a lot *more* health, until death do you part.

This is a lot more and a lot better than simply forcing yourself through a routine you think you have to do until you lose weight. To force (control) change takes energy; it fatigues you, and it's only a matter of time until you quit.

The components of your new approach to adding permanent exercise to your life are as follows:

1. *Safety*

What you do, how much you do it, when you do it, where you do it, with whom you do it, where you obtain your knowledge or training, how you progress, what factors influence your progress, and the equipment you use for exercising are all first considerations. If you're injured, you can't exercise at all. If you do it wrong, it won't work for you, and you will experience burnout.

A logical starting place is to assess your physical fitness level and basic health. The only time it may be safe to forego a general physical exam and physical fitness check before starting a new exercise routine would be if you have a personal family physician you see at least twice each year, and he or she gives you a green light with proper precautions; or if you are under 35 years old, have no personal or family history of cardio-respiratory, structural or alignment problems; no physical symptoms, have been living a healthful lifestyle, and are no more than twenty percent above your ideal weight. Everyone, whether or not they may exempt themselves from a physical evaluation prior to starting an exercise program, should use caution and patience in seeking a good level of exercise. Remember, you have the rest of your life to do it. Also, if you do have a weakness that needs to be protected, seek guidance and advice from an appropriate professional.

2. *Decide on a program.*

There are many options that will help you achieve a high level of health and fitness, with good weight balance. Some things you might ask about are:

- Do you have fundamental information about the activity?
- How convenient would it be for you?
- How much will it cost, and is it within your budget?
- Will it provide you with balanced exercise?
- How much variety does it have?
- Is it safe?
- Can you do it anywhere?
- Can you do it alone?

- How much equipment is needed?
- Most of all: are you interested in it?

You may want to consider planning several different activities to meet your changing needs and to help keep you from becoming bored or burning out. At the very least, it is advisable to make sure your exercise program is balanced. A good program will include stretching/limbering, aerobic, and contractual/firming activities. It will be progressive (can you do it more, longer, farther, etc. as your endurance builds?) up to the point where your ideal weight is achieved. You may want to consider some activities for your training program which you can do any time, any place. Other activities could be social or entertainment experiences and may be done only occasionally—you wouldn't count on them to meet any of your physical or health needs; but they would be for stimulation and entertainment. Some very active people use their training activities to support their sports or entertainment interests. Training activities should not put you in competition with other people—it is *your* optimum you are seeking. You only want to win for *you*. The effect of competition on weight problems will be discussed in other chapters. Some activities you may want to include are:

- Walking/hiking/jogging/running
- Biking/rowing/paddle boating
- Stair climbing/jumping rope
- Mountain climbing/skiing/skating
- Swimming/water aerobics
- Dance/aerobic low-impact with or without machines
- Yoga/tai chi
- Weight lifting
- Home exercise equipment, such as the Lifeline Gym (described below).

Try to put enough effort into these exercises so that your heart rate and respiration climb to a point where it is difficult to carry on a conversation.

This indicates that you are getting an aerobic workout. Many of these exercises can be done either indoors or outdoors; all can be done alone; many can be done either with or without machines or other equipment; most can be done at either low cost or at considerable expense; many are weight-bearing exercises; and some are for the lower body only.

3. *Determine what amount of exercise is right for you.*

How much to do certainly varies a great deal from person to person. A person who is generally in peak physical condition but who is ill with the flu or other short-term illness, should almost totally restrict exercise, as should someone who is in excellent general health (absence of illness) but who is not physically fit. Your age, the time of day, whether or not you are rested, if you have any injuries, your level of knowledge of the skills or movements involved in a particular activity, your frame of mind or mood, how repetitive the activity is, and how much interest you have in the activity are also variables that might influence how much exercise is appropriate on any given occasion.

If you are in good health but just starting an exercise program, it is most important to not overdo it. In the first place, you are trying to learn the movements correctly so that you don't end up stiff and unable to perform the next session. Going slowly while you determine your optimal starting point gives you time to make psychological adjustments. It is more important to want to repeat the exercise than to see how much you are able to do or how fast. Try starting with three exercise sessions each week and building up to five or six days each week while you are trying to lose weight, taking extra days off from time-to-time after you have achieved your weight goal. How much exercise you do during each session should also progress at an appropriate speed, until you reach your ideal weight.

It doesn't matter how little time you spend on your exercise routine to start with. Even five minutes is fine, as long as you add minutes each time you are able to do your routine easily. Work up to at least thirty minutes per session. For peak condition, work up to one hour. Distance and speed are variables of "how much" and can clearly affect the duration and difficulty. For the person losing weight, inappropriate speed, distance, and level of difficulty could bring greater possibilities of injury or psychological burnout. *Gradual* is the key here—and progressive and consistent are the goals. You can be a star tomorrow—but be a person who learns to love exercise first.

4. *Decide on the best time to exercise.*

When to do it includes some interesting options. Those who are most consistent with their routine tend to exercise in the morning. Morning exercisers are up to 75 percent more consistent than those choosing to exercise in the late afternoon or evening. On the other hand, those who exercise in the morning are more prone to injury. By afternoon or evening your connective tissue will be warmed and less tight. So, if you are searching for the best option, do an extra long warm-up and make morning exercise your first choice.

It seems even more important to be flexible with your routines. To become rigid or compulsive about when you do your exercise is going to set you up for stress, disappointment, and excuses for *not* doing your routine or burning out fast. This is why counting on set class times, counting on a friend, or counting on ideal weather tend to not work out. Always have options so you don't have to forego your exercise if one or more factors aren't favorable. Vacation time, business trips, or having guests in your home can also be excuses to procrastinate or quit. Routines are best when they can be kept throughout the year, no matter what the circumstance (except illness). It is very important to your own self-worth to see yourself make time available to do your routines, especially if you are stressed and short of time. This is the only way you will convince yourself of the importance of exercise and the fact that you are worth the trouble.

Seasons can also dictate a change in the time of day you choose to exercise. The number of hours of sunlight or daylight, the hours you work, and the type exercise you choose all have an effect on when you do your exercise. Be flexible, and be consistent—but don't be rigid! Fit exercise into your schedule when you can, but fit it in. Barring illness, missing more than twice a month can indicate you are having to push yourself to do it and are not giving it a true high priority. Let exercise be in your life!

5. *Select a place to exercise.*

Where to exercise includes many choices in the short term, but there is really only one choice for the long term. Today, the world is more geared to exercise than ever before. You can work out at commercial fitness centers, parks and recreation programs, private athletic clubs, tennis and swim clubs, community centers, school fitness centers and tracks, PAR courses, aerobic dance classes, hotel and airport workout rooms, corporate exercise programs, biking-, walking-, jogging-, hiking-, and cross-country skiing-clubs; rowing teams, water aerobic classes, neighborhood walking groups, hospital health promotion programs, athletic medicine clinics—and yes, even strolling around indoor shopping malls in the early hours is a way to exercise. All of these are good methods for you to get in shape.

These wonderful facilities and organizations are there for you, but they all have limitations, which mean you are not likely to stay with them for the rest of your life. There are many things to consider: cost, whether the facilities are available only at certain hours, how crowded they are, how good the instructors are, and whether it will become more of a social than a physical exercise. Or, sometimes, what you can do at a gym is limited, machines may be broken or overcrowded, or you feel like you're expected to keep pace with the others. . . The list of limitations goes on and on. None of them are as right for you as is the place where you already are. If you are going to exercise for life, you need to be able to do it at work, on the road and, especially, at home—the one place you are most apt to stay with it. All those other places are all right to use for variety, but don't count on them or come to feel you need them.

6. *Choose who to exercise with.*

There are not as many choices to make in terms of choosing exercise companions. Public or commercial places put you together with strangers, and that may or may not be a good motivator for you. Your friends and relatives may or may not be available to exercise with you. Sooner or later, the timing will be off. Some people may be able to afford a personal instructor/motivator. Some people follow television instructors. Some buy videos to use at home. Some have teachers at school or in the fitness centers, but the only person you can count on being there for sure is the person in the mirror.

Using well qualified instructors for a while to get you started on the right track is a wise idea. Instructors in books cannot see you and often leave out important, individualized information. Friends, spouse, kids, dogs, and neighbors are unlikely to have enough training to give you good information and will only motivate you in the short term, at best. If you have these people with you for awhile, enjoy them and get the most out of them, but, in the long run, plan to be your own main person in your own lifelong program—your own friend, teacher and, above all, motivator. I know people who have been waiting for years for their friend or spouse to exercise with them so they can get started. But this is your life, and nobody else's.

7. *Choose a source of information.*

Among your sources of information are books, magazines, videos, exercise facilitates, equipment manufacturers, and exercise specialists. Hopefully, your guide will not be your buddy who has been exercising just two weeks longer than you. The wrong advice could lead to injury, ineffective development, hard-to-break habits, a dislike for exercise, or quick burnout. I encourage you to read a book on the subject before you choose either an instructor or a facility from which to learn. Make sure the book, like the instructor or facility you eventually choose, has excellent credentials. Criteria should include information that has been well researched, recognition from known authorities in the field, academic credentials, ample, appropriate experience, and testimony by satisfied students or clients. If you have read up on the activity you wish to incorporate into your program, you will require less time with an instructor, you will learn faster, your questions will be fewer and more pertinent, and your expectations more realistic. Having a personal or classroom instructor provides you with someone who can observe you, guide you, correct you and help you to reach your potential. If your instructor works where you practice, you will have on-going attention and someone to help monitor your progress. Remember, just because an instructor is well-qualified in one activity, does not mean he or she is an expert in all exercise activities. Specialists can save you time, frustration, money, and possibly injury.

The best all-around help I have been able to find in my own community has been at the fitness center at my local community college. The instructors are highly trained in a variety of activities. They are there every day and have access to resources that supplement their personal skills. They make sure I am doing the exercises properly and safely, they help one another, and we have developed a personal working relationship—all at a very low cost.

8. *Measure your progress.*

Progress and factors that influence it are somewhat easily observed by yourself and others. A scale is unfortunately the one thing that most people trying to lose weight go by. If you are interested in long-term success and finding what your capabilities really are, a scale will be the least of your concerns. Even without a scale, your clothes and a mirror will tell you if you are the weight you want to be. A tape measure, like a scale, can be helpful, but what you see and how you feel tell you much more.

More difficult to observe, yet far more important, is what goes on underneath the skin and in your mind. What you really want to lose is *fat*, not just weight. *Fat loss* can't be measured by a scale, tape measure, or visual observation. Weight loss without exercise can easily lead to a higher percentage of your remaining body weight being composed of fat as opposed to muscle and water. Without exercise, even bone density can become less. If you squeeze someone who has an average height-to-weight ratio but has done little or no exercise, they could feel like mush. As you may know, muscle is denser and heavier than fat. It is made up mostly of water and protein. Protein and the carbohydrates that fuel muscle burn two and a half times as fast as fat. So, if you are not exercising while losing meaningful amounts of weight, the muscle loss will be much greater than you want. The majority of diets end up being diuretic diets where more water is lost than anything else. The best weight loss is fat loss.

There are a couple of good methods for assessing how much of your weight loss is fat. One is a body composition analyzer, an electronic instrument that works much like sonar in ships. Input your correct gender, weight, height, and age and, in a few seconds, it can give you an assessment of your weight broken down into water, muscle, and fat percentages. Weight loss facilities and fitness centers now commonly have either this type of body composition analyzer, or they use hand-held calipers to measure percent of body fat. Calipers work like the pinch test with your fingers, measuring the fat in a one-inch pinch at key sites on the body. A mathematical formula can give you a fairly close measurement. Probably the most accurate means of measuring body fat, if done correctly, is water weighing, usually done only at a hospital, university, or sports medicine facility. It is much more expensive, takes much longer, with the added inconvenience of having to don a bathing suit, hold your breath, and be dunked under water for longer than most people like.

It should also be remembered that exercise may bring enough muscle gain while you are burning fat that weight loss seems slower than you would expect at times. A tape measure can usually alleviate concern if your measurements improve even though your weight goes up or stays the same.

A physical fitness check can give you valuable measurements of your success, and good fitness centers will make sure you complete the tests before allowing you to exercise. You can often find testing facilities at community college and university facilities. While they may also be offered by heart clinics, the prices they charge can be substantial.

A fitness check usually includes:

1. Treadmill EKG (electrocardiogram), or step test: Measures heart-beat, pulse, and blood pressure. With the step test, blood pressure is measured separately.

2. Pulmonary check: Measures lung capacity for delivery of oxygen.

3. Body composition: Measures percentages of body mass made up of muscle, water, and fat.

4. Flexibility: Measures the extent you can stretch, pointing out potential injury sites for different activities.

5. Strength/poser: Measures safe lifting range or other activities requiring this capacity.

6. Endurance: Measures how long you can safely stay with an activity.

7. Blood analysis: Measures the composition of the blood and its capacity to carry oxygen. Not all fitness checks include the blood

analysis, due to cost and other restrictive administrative controls. The twenty most commonly measured blood factors and how to interpret the results of your profile are included as Appendix B.

Other measurements of your exercise progress are taken by yourself and who observe you and are more subjective. They would include things like increased energy level, your endurance on hard days, your sense of well-being, your attitudes, how you handle stress and depression, your sexual appetite, your coloring, humor, and, with some people, possibly even your resistance to colds and flu. What is most important to long-term success, though, is your growing appreciation for your exercise routines as seen in your attitudes about doing it, the priority it takes when you're pressed for time, how you talk to other people about it, how much you seek new challenges in your exercise program and, most of all, how consistently you look forward to doing it, miss it when you don't do it, and whether you turn to exercise or food when you are distressed.

How well you progress in your physical development, the appreciation you hold for exercise, and how long you continue your program are important factors that can be influenced by many other things, some of which you may not have thought of:

- Approval and support from important people in your life
- Your nutritional habits
- Work habits and requirements
- Travel and adjustments for it
- Social and religious involvements and adjustments
- Involvement/and modeling attitudes within your family
- Where you live (climate/community).

The list can go on and on. Progress may be slower or faster, easier or harder, depending on these variables.

9. *Select the proper clothing and shoes.*

Clothing and shoes are not always necessary when you are exercising in the privacy of your own home. Exercising in the nude can be a wonderful, freeing experience if you have comfortable rugs or mats and you either live alone or have a partner who appreciates the fun or values the non-conformity of it. The views and poses are unusual, and if you try it once, you may want to do it again. This is certainly not a requirement, or for everybody, but, remember, changing yourself means not only establishing exercise routines, but also changing some of the attitudes that may have held you back. Relax!

If you plan to exercise outdoors and in public places, the right clothes and shoes will not only provide modesty but also protect you from the elements and foot damage. Clothes can also help you look good, which is part of the reason most people exercise in the first place. Practical, colorful, attractive clothing and shoes can also stimulate you, simply because you know you look good and color enlivens us. If, however, your main concern with clothing is for social reasons or to look sexy, your motivation priorities may benefit from some re-examination. Bright, luminescent colors are practical at night when jogging or riding a bike on the side of the road. Tight fitting materials can keep you from getting hung up in equipment or causing other accidents, yet provide excellent freedom of movement. Gortex and other relatively new materials do an excellent job of keeping your muscles warm (without overheating), removing the excess water from your skin, and promoting evaporation, which protects against such things as hypothermia in cool weather and chafing in warm weather. Your body burns calories to keep a stable temperature in cold weather, and flushes water in warm weather. Avoid overdressing in either type of weather just to cover up unwanted pounds.

Nothing is more important to lifelong exercise than your feet, knees and legs. Having the right footwear for the right activity can go a long way toward keeping you injury free, enjoying your workouts, and reaching your optimal performance levels. This is especially true for the overweight person. The right fit for width and length, along with sufficient support to keep your foot stable but flexible, with ample cushioning to absorb the pounding is a tall order. Unfortunately, all of these requirements in a single shoe that has good durability can be costly, especially when it is recommended that new shoes be purchased every three months or two hundred miles, whichever comes first. With prices ranging from $30 to $150 per pair, it is helpful to find a discount store that carries your brand. Wearing worn out or inadequate footwear could, on the other hand, lead to expensive medical bills and considerable pain. Seek out the best personal guidance possible to make sure you select the right footwear for the right sport. Some possible sources of guidance are podiatrists, training books and manuals on the activity you're interested in, specialty magazines covering your activities—such as *Runner's World* or organization newsletters. Some stores that specialize in carrying a wide selection of footwear for all popular exercise activities in a good range of prices will have at least one sales clerk who has a fundamental knowledge of the shoes, but not necessarily with your feet, knees and legs. If you have special problems with these areas, I strongly suggest you see a podiatrist, orthopedic or athletic medicine doctor who exercises regularly.

Special gear such as orthotics (foot supports) should be especially made for your feet. Waist belts, wrist supports and headbands to keep the sweat out of your eyes can be helpful, too.

10. *Choose the right equipment.*

Equipment is essential to any well balanced personal exercise/fitness program. As I stated before, fitness is not just weight loss, it is fat loss. Firming, shaping, and aerobic exercise, along with stretching and limbering are all necessary. It is important to be able to exercise where and when you want. Instead of being able to find convenient excues *not* to exercise, give yourself convenient excuses *to* exercise.

It is not my intent here to discourage the use or membership in public or private fitness center. As I mentioned earlier, I am a member of one myself. For the training I get there, the social aspects of working out with other like-minded people, and even as a place to discuss business, it has clear advantages. Also, I could never afford, nor do I have space for all that beautiful, chrome-plated equipment. However, if you are serious about exercise, plan to exercise for a lifetime, and see sports only as another reason to have a regular exercise program, then if you restrict yourself to a certain place, specific hours or require the presence of other people, your chances of continuing to exercise on a regular basis are greatly reduced. These restrictions are also a statement about your commitment.

When you are without special exercise equipment, workouts can also be done by using your body as a weight, walking, jogging, or improvising with chairs, suitcases, door frames, etc. But, it is much harder to get a full, balanced workout, and, psychologically, it is not nearly as motivating as being able to do your own familiar routine. The longer you exercise, the more refined your skills, knowledge and sensitivities become. You know when you've had a good session and how to get at those places that need more work. So, your appreciation of good, versatile, durable equipment grows along with you physical development.

Because weight loss is a very personal thing, there are many reasons why your best chance of keeping those extra pounds off is through setting up your own program. Being able to exercise on your own is a key aspect of your main goals of fitness and health (including a balanced height to weight ratio). There are many optional pieces of equipment that can give you a workout at home, but most of them have drawbacks, such as the price, which can be in the thousands of dollars. Some equipment is large, takes up a great deal of space, and has to stay put because it is so heavy to move. Many expensive pieces of equipment only work one or a few parts of the body (i.e., treadmills). Some have many moving parts that tend to break down over time or need regular maintenance. Other equipment is dangerous to use and slow in moving from one exercise movement to another, such as free weights which have to be moved between exercise sessions and can damage floors, carpets, furniture, or even yourself if you should drop them or lift them in the wrong way. Worst of all, most of this equipment for home use restricted to just that: "home use." You can't take it with you. In general, the equipment that can be taken with you has always been awkward to pack, easily broken, poorly made, difficult to use, or, again, too limited in regard to what you can do with it.

I do recommend that you buy personal use exercise equipment not only for the reasons I've mentioned regarding your best chance for long-term success with your weight, but also because it is essential to stay with your exercise for life in order to give yourself the best chance to enjoy optimal health and well-being. It is unlikely that the average person on the move in this busy world will continue to use a facility or group with consistency over the long haul.

Because of my keen interest in and dedication to consistent exercise in my own life, it is not surprising that I've found an answer to the question, "what personal equipment is available that meets all the needs of the average person for weight loss and beyond?"

About twenty years ago, I was traveling a great deal in my work and it seemed as though I just could not get to the fitness spa I was using at the time. I wasn't home to use my own equipment, and most of the portable equipment I tried to take with me was far too limited. What I found on the road was very hit or miss, and usually with my schedule, I just wasn't getting my exercise routine in. Then one day on "Hour Magazine," a television show hosted by Gary Collins, there appeared a guest with a wondrous little two pound bag of exercise equipment which would provide me with the means to achieve all the benefits of exercise I could expect to find in a complete fitness center.

As I watched its inventor, Bobby Hinds, demonstrate it, I knew it provided for all my needs and more. The name of the product was "Lifeline Gym," and it was portable, light-weight, and disassembled into a small carrying case. It could be adapted to almost any environment, any type of exercise movement, or any person. I could workout in my hotel room, my office, my home, even on a camping trip—anywhere I could find ten square feet of space. I could make every exercise movement that I did in the spa, I could have any amount of resistance, I could change exercises rapidly. There were no heavy weights to do damage to me or property. It was extremely durable, with no mechanical parts to break down. The cost was very low, the equipment required little or no storage space and could be put out of sight easily.

Probably the part I liked best was that it could provide an aerobic workout as well as aid in muscle development, toning and shaping. It was so simple and adaptable to individual needs that anybody could use it—from a little elderly lady to the most powerful professional athlete. It came with what was described as a "treadmill belt," only it was like no treadmill I had ever seen. It allowed the user to move around from side-to-side, or walk or run backward or forward. It didn't require that I hold on to bars to avoid falling down, and it even gave met he freedom to answer the phone or change channels on television without skipping a step.

Twenty years later, this product is still on the market, only now it is even better. It is called "The Lifeline Gym" and you can order it by calling 1-800-553-6633. Tell them your age, size, and your needs, and they'll mail you a gym that is just right for you. If you prefer to write, mail your request to: Lifeline International, Inc., 3201 Syene Rd., Madison, WI 53713.

11. *Establish harmony between mind and body.*

Body-mind harmony is essential to the lifelong enjoyment of exercise as an integral part of your lifestyle. To have harmony between your mind and body, is to be balanced and calm, with your energy focused. At that point, no struggle exists within yourself, nor between you and the ground, gravity, the air, objects, other people, or any other part of your environment. When the process of movement is done for the inner joy, and not just the pride and ego satisfaction that you feel after it is over, no question exists whether you will or won't exercise. It doesn't make you a good or bad person, it simply is part of who you are.

Adding exercise permanently to your life usually means something else may have to be reduced, changed, or eliminated. If you let go of some self-defeating activities in favor of exercise, you have an even better chance that your restructured priorities will last. If, like Louise, for example, you let go of Friday evening out with the girls (a fattening supper and a few drinks at the bar), you may miss the old times for awhile until you make new friends at the fitness center and start getting in shape. As you establish friendships with new people who share a common interest in healthful living, some of your old friends may drift out of your life. Yet others may join you at the fitness center.

Changing one aspect of your life will, in some way, affect other aspects of your life. At first, it does make it hard, but because it is hard, when you are successful in making a change you will be more impressed with the changes you've made and your self-esteem will rise even higher.

As with dieting, "gradual" is the operative word in change. Your body changes are gradual so you don't injure yourself, get stiff and uncomfortable, or suffer psychological burnout. Changing gradually also give you time to make mental adjustments that allow you to find the joy in your changes.

There are many, varied approaches to developing a true commitment to exercise. The following are just a few examples.

- Frequently adding variety in time, place, and activity helps. The same basic movements can be done in many ways.

- Exercise with a partner or a group, or exercise alone.

- Keep expectations for yourself minimal. Make decisions as you go.

- Avoid comparisons or competition. It only leads to burnout and emotional stress.

- Learn to focus on what is happening within yourself; be sensitive to your physical and emotional self.

- Fantasize/imagine the present; and envision the path you wish to walk in the future.

- Involve yourself with your environment (i.e., notice the air, birds and natural sounds).

- Practice meditation and/or self-hypnosis.

- Let go of mental conflicts (struggling with yourself about whether or not you will exercise today).

- Strive for mastery, taking a regular practice and turning it into a discipline, helping yourself to let go of your need for instant gratification until you look forward to practicing it.

All the above suggestions may be helpful in bringing about a permanent incorporation of exercise in your lifestyle. But probably none is as important as the last approach: mastery.

The idea of mastery certainly applies beautifully to the role of exercise in effective weight change efforts and, in addition, once the concept is understood it is easy to see how it applies to all other aspects of self-change and dealing with the stress-bound world in which we find ourselves.

Dr. George Leonard is the person responsible for bringing this profound concept to my attention in his recently-published book entitled *Mastery*. some of his earlier writings, which include *The Silent Pulse*, *The Transformation*, and *The Ultimate Athlete*, have also contributed to my improved understanding of self-efficacy.

In Dr. Leonard's view of mastery, the aspects most relevant to developing intrinsic change are:

- Letting go of our addiction to the quick fix and our never-ending, never-fulfilling quest for a series of climactic moments, as demonstrated in thel popular view of nymphomania.

- Finding a natural rhythm or harmony of life instead of attempting to force, control, or contain behavior.

- Returning again and again to a discipline or task, even when you appear to be going nowhere.

- Living more fully in the present moment with keener awareness and sensitivity to your world.

- Shifting personal values and beliefs from hyped-up, high-fat materialism, to how it feels physically and emotionally to be alive.

- Practicing (like a ritual) not to achieve a goal (although goals will be a by-product), but to define who we are. Practice is not done rigidly but consistently, convincing us of our own trustworthiness and value to ourselves—it is our inner security.

- Having a vision (a direction)—we must decide which way to head. Our intention—even if we do not arrive where we headed—determines where we end up. We need a vision which isn't a continuous series of highs. Learning what is satisfying is *climbing* to the high instead of buying addictive food highs.

- Becoming aware that learning includes both going up and down—a little less down after each new higher up and spending a lot of time on plateaus with some climaxes along the way, with no real end, just continual growth and learning. The climaxes are by-products of staying in practice, and you never know for sure when they will come. (Twenty years ago, I stumbled for awhile over Dr. Leonard's point, and then made up a saying from it that I now strive to live by: "Seek not in vain for happiness, for it shall come to those worthy of being found.")

- Practicing in a centered (balanced) way; unrushed and focused on the movements, not the outcome. Knowing the path on which you walk.

- Making a connection between the practice of mastery and positive social transformation. Focus on the moment, and the result will be positive global awareness.

Dr. Leonard uses the martial art discipline of aikido to achieve the base from which transformation can come, but anything from gardening to meditation to stamp collecting to art will do. It is something you do on a regular basis, not casually, as long as you don't do it to win prizes. The mastery is really of yourself, and the process is a path you walk by which you know yourself. My years of morning yoga, aerobics and weight lifting have truly let me know who I am, just as Louise is learning to know herself and just as you can learn to know yourself. We are all in a constant, unending state of becoming. We will always be able to find something new and more stimulating from the routines of what we do. Choose something and do it, and do it, and do it, without expecting anything more than you get from doing it over and over, and the rewards will come.

The psychology of exercise is getting your mind into the physical movements—not the payoff (i.e., being thin). We all have an athlete in us, and we will discover that athlete only after we quit searching for him or her and have instead realized the joy in accomplishing the difficult.

Chapter 9

THE 5-PLUS CLUB

A Profile for Success

*A*s difficult as it is for individuals to lose weight and to change their eating, exercise and overall health patterns, many people are victorious in the struggle. Identifying what characteristics those who are successful share can lead to a greater understanding of how to achieve one's own weight loss goals.

In addition, many myths circulate about those who can and those who cannot lose weight and successfully maintain the weight loss. For instance, childhood obesity means lifelong weight problems; the more weight loss programs you have participated in, the less chance for success you have; etc. However, the truth is not as limiting as these myths lead us to believe. There are basically no physical or circumstantial reasons why anybody who is open to the possibility cannot successfully lose and maintain weight loss. On the other hand, there are indeed commonalities among those individuals who are successful. Interestingly, these characteristics depend more on attitude, approach and method than on external and historical circumstances.

In 1990, I conducted my own research study/survey of thirty individuals who had lost 20 pounds or more and had kept if off for five years or longer. To these individuals, I bestowed membership in what I call the "5-Plus Club." The conclusions presented in this chapter arise from the interviews I conducted with members of the 5-Plus Club, and they verify and add to earlier data gathered by Dr. Stanton Peele in his book *Diseasing of America*

(Lexington Books, 1989). This chapter will review what characteristics contribute to successful, long-term weight loss by pointing out the traits common among the 5-Plus Club members. It also discusses and debunks some of the popular myths about why many people cannot lose weight and/or cannot keep it off once they have lost it.

When I conducted my research, Louise had not qualified to become a part of this group, but only because it had not yet been five years since she successfully lost her weight. In the meantime, she had developed or was in the process of developing many of the same characteristics and behaviors of the 5-Plus Club members, including acquiring ever-growing confidence as her change developed.

Most of the thousands of research studies that have been done on the topic of weight loss consider weight problems from a historical, physiological, sociological, or psychological point of view. These studies are often subtly biased with an attitude that something needs to be *cured* in these individuals—as if weight problems are an illness. In other words, the preconception is that intervention and treatment are believed to be the only means of recovery. Very few researchers have made any attempt to examine the possibility that weight problems can be resolved by individuals on their own. Yet my study shows quite the opposite. It is very possible.

In the past, very few studies, if any, actually examined or even considered those people who have lost a good deal of weight and kept it off beyond the time during which 90 to 98 percent of people who have lost weight gain it back. The few studies that were done looked at other compulsive behaviors, such as drinking, smoking, gambling, etc., along with overeating. For the most part, these studies have not considered what factors these groups may have in common and which enable them to reach and sustain their goals.

Knowing what commonly has contributed to the long-term success of others does not mean everyone else who follows suit will also succeed. Nor does the availability of this information assure that many people will make use of it. However, it does imply that whoever examines this information has some potentially powerful new choices available to them. Providing this type of information may positively influence previously negative attitudes, or at least it may save individuals a great deal of money and encourage avoidance of practices that may negatively affect one's health.

Weight loss appears to be a choice, hard or not so hard, rather than the result of some other factor or combination of factors. It does not seem to have a single cause, nor a single cure. It does not appear to be a disease, nor does it appear to be devoid of socio/cultural influences. Those who have succeeded in achieving and maintaining weight loss are far fewer in number than those who have lost and regained the weight. However, looking closely at the means, methods, and myths involved may start a new belief that obesity is primarily a psychological matter rather than an illness or a predetermined, genetic condition that makes the difference.

My study of members of the 5-Plus Club included only a small statistical sample (i.e., 30 research subjects), but the results still raise strong questions regarding old beliefs about how people lose weight and keep it off. And, certainly, the study points out the urgent need for large-scale studies to examine the questions raised by the results. The findings are only raw numbers and percentages, but, without a doubt, these findings challenge old beliefs.

All the subjects in my study were found through referral from friends, a feature article in the *Arizona Republic*, and a local radio talk show. One-on-one interviews were conducted, and clear, specific responses were sought.

The 5-Plus Club members ranged in age from 20 to 77 years, with a mean age of 43. Sixty-seven percent of the group surveyed was female. The amount of weight they had lost ranged from 20 to 170 lbs., with a mean of 43 lbs. The time they had kept the weight off ranged from the minimum of 5 years to a high of 40 years, with a mean of 14.5 years.

The Interview Process

Structured interviews were used as the means of investigation. The questions were read to the subject so that follow-up and clarification were possible. A model questionnaire was used with several people before the final questionnaire was prepared. Most interviews, which ranged from 30 to 60 minutes in length, were conducted in person, either at my office or in public places such as a community college, and a few were conducted at the participant's place of business. If none of these options were available, the interview was conducted by telephone. No reward was offered as an incentive to participate in the interview. At the end of the interview I offered to provide the interviewees with a copy of any future publication of the data.

The subjects were proud of their achievements and seemed to enjoy the interview. Only information collected by request, in a pleasant and grateful manner, was utilized. No debate or discussion about right or wrong was brought into the interview. I used positive reinforcement of the participants' successes, and I shared personal information about my own life as a means of relaxing the subjects.

WEIGHT LOSS STATISTICS

The number of years members of this group had maintained their weight loss ranged from a minimum of 5 years to a maximum of 40 years. The average (mean) for the group was 14.5 years of having maintained at least a 20-pound weight loss. It should be noted that not all of the subjects sustained 100 percent of their original weight loss, and not all of them reached their ideal weight.

Maintained weight loss for the 5-Plus Club ranged from 20 to 170 pounds, with the average being 43 pounds. After five years, the percentage of weight loss retained varied from 36 percent to 100 percent, with the largest percentage of subjects (73.3 percent) having kept off 100 percent of the weight they lost.

Three people maintained 36 to 50 percent of their weight loss, and four held at 70 to 76 percent of their original weight loss. Nineteen of the 22 who had retained a 100 percent weight loss were at their ideal weight. Reaching the ideal weight may be connected with how much of a continuing mental/emotional struggle goes on within the individual. To be considered at an ideal weight, the participant must have been within five pounds of their ideal weight. This margin allowed for normal daily water weight fluctuations.

Fourteen (46.6 percent) of the participants in this study had reached their ideal weight and maintained 100 percent of their weight loss. They were comfortable with the way they ate and exercised, and enjoyed staying at their ideal weight without worry about regaining the extra pounds.

For another 14 participants, it continued to be a daily struggle. In this group, some had not reached their ideal weight or had not maintained 100 percent of their original weight loss. For those going through their daily struggle, it is an inner conflict between logic and emotions—trying not to always think about food, resenting exercise, or constantly having to choose between fattening or healthful foods. It is a one-day-at-a time effort to maintain "control." Those who were not struggling found a harmony between the emotions and the nutrition their bodies require. Two of the 5-Plus Club members have had *less* of a struggle since reaching and maintaining their ideal weight. For these two, it was a continual process of learning to deal with their emotions and the pressures of their everyday lives.

Onset of Weight Problems

The onset of weight problems among the research group was fairly well balanced, with 33.3 percent starting during childhood, 43.3 percent during the teen years (usually at the onset of puberty), and 23.3 percent during early adult years (most commonly in the mid to early twenties). These statistics do pose some questions about the nature/nurture aspect of etiology and change.

Educational Background of Participants

As a whole, the 5-Plus Club is highly educated, with 86.6 percent having at least one or more years of college. A bachelor's degree was most common among the group members (46.6 percent), with 16.6 percent holding master's degrees and 10 percent having doctorates. All participants had completed high school, and those who had stopped formal education at the 12th grade were highly self-educated and very bright. It appears likely that general education level may have some bearing on self-esteem and self-efficacy; although, in looking at chronically overweight people in general, or those who use commercial programs, the individuals in this study represented a wide range of education levels.

In the general population, lower socioeconomic groups (to include lower education levels) have a higher percentage of weight problems. Many of those in the poorer groups spend money they can't afford or go into debt to pay for commercial programs to give what looks like a balance to the socioeconomic groups enrolled in commercial weight loss programs.

Personality Traits of Research Subjects

As a group, the 5-Plus Club consisted chiefly of outgoing persons, with 76.6 percent of them identifying themselves as comfortable social mixers. This, again, may indicate a higher confidence level than the average overweight person. In a stressful world where so much of that stress comes from social interaction, and so much inappropriate eating comes from stress, social factors (self-esteem, educational level, socioeconomic level) may all tie together to influence self-efficacy.

Previous Weight Loss Efforts

Only seven of the 5-Plus Club members did not seek help in their original attempts to lose weight. Most of these people were able to maintain long-term weight loss with their first effort, even though they had been overweight for some time. One of these seven had gained back all but 36 percent of what he originally lost and experienced on-going inner conflict.

Among the other 23 (76.6 percent) participants, outside help was sought one or more times, each time resulting in their regaining what was lost—and often more. Only four people in the total group had received outside assistance with their long-term weight loss. Three of these regained part of the weight they originally lost, and all four of them still experienced a mental struggle. The vast majority of the group (26 subjects, or 86.6 percent) were not able to successfully maintain their weight loss until they achieved it on their own.

From this study, it appears that self-direction is extremely important to successful, long-term weight loss and that receiving outside assistance is likely to be counterproductive.

Binge eating, which is eating large amount of foods at one single time (often within a 20 minute period), and purging, which is the use of laxatives and forced regurgitation prior to digestion, are both common behaviors exhibited by people who utilize commercial weight loss programs. There may be a greater prevalance of binge eating. With fasting programs, binge eating after the fast is extremely common. Thirty-three percent of the 5-Plus Club had binged prior to their successful last weight-loss effort, and 20 percent had purged. In each case, the purging was usually only done for a short time. Within the group as a whole, no binge eating or purging had taken place since their successful long-term effort.

Many possibilities could be explored concerning why the binge eating and purging stopped, and it is only a guess to assume that health and self-responsibility have become more prominent motivators when long-term success is achieved. Yo-yoing two or more times took place with 43.3 percent of the 5-Plus Club prior to their long-term success. Yo-yoing after long-term success was reported by only one member. After as long as five years, it seems unlikely that members of this group would believe in any radical weight loss methods, and they probably have a greater commitment to continue with what has brought them long-term success and, along with it, greater confidence.

Dietary Changes among 5-Plus Club Members

All the members of the 5-Plus Club substantially reduced their fat intake, and 46 percent of them became vegetarians. At the time of the interview, only one of them was a vegan vegetarian (no animal products). The remainder of the vegetarians eat either dairy or poultry products, or a combination of these.

Relationship Changes among 5-Plus Club Members

Compared with the time when they were overweight, the stability of the home life of 5-Plus Club members improved by 33.3 percent. The percentage who had been abused as children was 16.6. Verbal abuse was most common; however, there was some physical abuse and one person had been sexually abused. For most of the total group, bringing their weight into balance was just part of balancing out the whole of their lives.

Stress and Emotional Eating Responses among 5-Plus Club Members

Eating in response to their emotions was one of the most common characteristics of the 5-Plus Club members at the time they were overweight. Twenty-six (86.6 percent) felt that eating was a way of dealing with their feelings, and this had become a conditioned response to almost any type of stress, negative or positive. At the time my research with these individuals was conducted, (5 years or more following their weight loss) emotional eating was reported by only 33.3 percent of the group, and everyone had either developed or was in the process of developing new ways of dealing with stress. Although some emotional eating still occurred, it was much less frequent—as were the urges to do it—and when it happened, it was managed much more effectively and lasted much shorter.

The amount of stress experienced by this group had also been reduced a great deal. *Remember, think of stress/distress as a person's perceived ability to deal effectively with whatever challenges are confronting him or her.* At the time of their peak weights, 96.6 percent of the 5-Plus Club members felt they were experiencing high levels of stress, or anxiety. When they were interviewed, 33.3 percent felt they were under high levels of stress, but how they were handling the stress was much improved. Six percent felt their stress levels were medium, and 46.6 percent now feel their stress levels were low. Even though some of the reduced stress was likely to be circumstantial, a change in self-perception is also certain to influence the level of stress, especially after a successful, self-directed weight balance effort.

The Role of Perfectionism in Weight Control

Perfectionism, quality of home life, stress levels, and emotional eating can all be tied together, so it is not surprising that 93.3 percent of the 5-Plus Club members saw themselves (as did others) as perfectionists at the time of their highest weight. At the time of my study, the number of subjects that thought of themselves as perfectionists was reduced to 50 percent, while

46.6 percent of the group felt they were significantly less perfectionist, and one man felt that he had never been a perfectionist.

Perfectionism is frequently a result of unstable homes. It creates a greater likelihood of high levels of stress and, in turn, contributes to emotional eating. Also, control is a common need of perfectionists, and food is one area of the perfectionist's life that he or she can control. Furthermore, overeating becomes a good arena in which to rebel against one's own perfectionism in a passive-aggressive way.

Perfectionism, control, and a need to rebel seem to be interrelated. Of the 5-Plus Club members, 76.6 percent indicated they had been, or continued to be, rebellious. Because dieters often have been people-pleasers, putting others' needs ahead of their own, they strive to be right by trying to be in control. Therefore, to submit to something like a structured diet or group plan brings up resentment and rebellious behavior which is often pushed into the subconscious.

Physical Problems and Weight Control

Nine members of my research group indicated that they had some physical problem that contributed to their weight problem. Although six of the nine had at some time been diagnosed with a thyroid condition, all but one had long since stopped taking medication for it, and at this time wondered if they had ever really had a thyroid disorder. One member reported a heart condition that had been successfully treated surgically, one was taking steroids for an asthmatic condition, and one suffered from severe water retention. At the time of the interview, all of these disorders had been cleared up, possibly as a result of the changes the subjects had made in lifestyle and increased self-efficacy.

The Relationship between Self-Esteem and Weight

How much a person is hugged and assured they are loved certainly ties into the level of self-esteem and self-worth, which of course is tied into perfectionism, stress levels, and emotional eating. Just on the basis of raw numbers, it appears that the tie-in is an important factor. During their obese years, only a third of my research group felt loved and reported receiving hugs on a regular basis. At the time of the study, 66.6 percent felt they got ample verbal affirmation and touching, and even those who did not, for the most part, felt loved. As the title of this book implies, food may often be substituted for the real thing.

The Impact of Knowledge

Knowledge of nutrition, exercise, and methods of weight loss does play some role in long-term success, but it does not seem to be a mandatory prerequisite. Prior to their successful efforts, 46.6 percent of the group had little knowledge of nutrition, but by the time they had reached five or more years of balanced weight, only one person in the group felt he lacked basic knowledge about food as it relates to fat. Knowledge of exercise increased even more, with only 43.4 percent of the group considering themselves aware of proper exercise at the time they began their final weight loss effort, while 100 percent of them now felt very knowledgeable about which exercises worked for them.

Information about various weight loss programs and methods was another story. It should be remembered that 76.6 percent of this group had tried various programs without success prior to attempting weight loss on their own. Also, 73.3 percent of them came from families with histories of weight problems. Before making the final weight loss attempt, 86.6 percent of the group felt they had ample information about commercial weight loss programs and other methods to lose weight at the time of the interview. Only one felt she had little information on programs or methods. The idea of needing or seeking help for weight problems was much more common than learning about nutrition and exercise as a solution. This fact (the successful group had much information about programs and little about nutrition and exercise) also suggests that when people decide to change their weight and lifestyle on their own, they will seek out the information they need as they need it, and that information is easily available from a wide variety of mostly free resources.

Substance Use/Abuse and Weight

Few members of the 5-Plus Club came from families of chemical abusers. Three came from homes where one parent was alcoholic, and one member came from a home where both parents abused alcohol and drugs. Fifty percent of the members became users of alcohol, but were not addicted, and after changing their lifestyles, only two remained users (but not abusers). Ten members of the group started out as smokers—about the same as the national average—and two remain smokers today.

Just utilizing this small study, it would appear that use of addictive substances, or having addicted parents, does not meaningfully impact the ability of an individual to change his or her weight or lifestyle. It does, however, raise questions about dependent personalities and the influence parents have on making it more difficult for their children to live healthful lifestyles.

Depression and Weight

Depression had been common among the group, with 73.3 percent of the subjects reporting they have had feelings of depression that were, for the most part, related to their weight. A little more than 23 percent still had recurring, but manageable, bouts of depression. It is interesting to note that most of those still experiencing depression were also still struggling emotionally with their food choices and/or had not retained 100 percent of their weight loss. One subject was ending a marriage of 14 years and was having to move to Alaska to secure adequate employment. It did not appear as though many in this group became obese as a result of their depression.

The Heredity Factor

It is clear, with this group at least, that having one or both overweight parents does not mean the child need be overweight. Twenty-two of the 30 came from families where either one or both of the parents had a weight problem. Sixty percent of the time, it was the mother, and a third of the time it was the father. A third of the group was currently married to a spouse who had a weight problem. It seems to be increasingly clear that unwanted weight, and whether or not we can keep it off once we lose it, is a personal choice, loaded with possibilities, blame, or avoidance.

The Motivation for Weight Loss

The members' motivations for losing weight and maintaining the weight loss can be divided into five main categories, with two of the motivating factors being most notable. These results agree nicely with the findings of many previous studies.

1. *Appearance.* The number one motivation at the start of the weight loss effort, and during younger years, was appearance (43.3 percent).

2. *Health.* After five years or more of maintained weight loss, the primary motivation was health (56.6 percent).

3. *Social Approval.* This ranged from approximately 17 percent to 0 percent within the 5-Plus Club, indicating a decrease in the need to meet social expectations or in having met them.

4. *Self-esteem.* Self-esteem was a motivating factor for only 10 to 6.6 percent of the subjects. Many did not identify with the need to improve self-esteem, and yet after the weight loss and a demonstrated ability to keep it off, those in the 5-Plus Club had elevated self-esteem levels more for their self-directed efforts than their weight loss.

5. *Other:* This section includes desire for better sex, more energy, fitness, and/or an ability to be more active. Each of these was cited by one member of the 5-Plus Club as their motivation for losing weight.

All of the members of the 5-Plus Club demonstrated at least some, if not a great deal of, intrinsic motivation for weight loss. Most of the people who had reached their ideal weight and maintained it with little or no mental struggle about their lifestyle could be considered primarily intrinsically motivated. The other members of the group were at various levels of developing intrinsic motivation, but still had, to some degree, an external focus on environmental direction and rewards. Some had yet to develop the personal insight which might justify a few counseling sessions with an existential counselor (one who believes and facilitates the idea that we all are free to determine much of our life outcomes) of their choice. People are motivated to procrastinate, and these motivations need to be looked into as much as, if not more than, the motivations to change.

The Relationship between Career and Weight

More than half the 5-Plus Club members stated they were satisfied with their careers, even when they attributed a good deal of their stress to their job. Twenty percent were dissatisfied, and 23.3 percent were neutral—that is, they fluctuated between satisfaction and dissatisfaction. Those in the neutral group did not find a great deal of meaning and purpose in their work, but were stimulated from time to time. Work is such a major part of adult life and self-image that this subject needs a great deal more investigation as to the impact it has on weight. We do know that work can be a major source of stress and, therefore, it can impact eating and exercise behavior. However, many people who learn how to handle stress with productive outlets and support systems no longer find food a necessary tool for coping.

Using Food as a Substitute for Sex

Using food as a substitute for sexual release is more common than you might imagine. Over half (53.3 percent) of the 5-Plus Club members felt they had used food in this manner in the past, and at the time of the study, 23.3 percent said they still did, although usually without being aware at the time they're doing it. Because relationships tend to wax and wane while the biological cycle that may cause sexual tension continues when a person is good health—whether or not the person is in a relationship that provides for regular release of sexual tension—food is a likely substitute for sexual pleasure. Interestingly, a study by Dr. Anna Rose of the University of Pennsylvania Children's Hospital observes that sex and drug cravings are seated in the same part of the brain. It is possible that food cravings are also located in the same area. We seek are less likely to seek food substitations when we like who we are and when we have good relationships established. If we had a greater awareness of our own sexuality and less inhibition regarding auto-eroticism, then this would be a minor difficulty. However, this area is sensitive for some, and one must be cautious when asking questions concerning another's sex life.

The Importance of an Emotional Support System

One thing at which this group has, as a whole, done exceptionally well, is gaining emotional support and release. All but one group member used at least one means of emotional release, while 83.3 percent used two or more means of release or support. Three used exercise only, and one used religion only. Included as one or more of the support mechanisms, in order of popularity, were the following:

1. Exercise   73.3 percent

2. Spouse   46.6 percent

3. Friends   46.6 percent

4. Parents/siblings   33.3 percent

5. Religion   30 percent

6. Books   26.6 percent

7. Meditation   13.3 percent

8. Group therapy   10 percent

9. Eating   10 percent

Other means, including journal keeping, children, housework, golf, yoga, parties, alcohol, kneading dough, and listing to the radio were each used by one person in the group.

When family members or friends were used for support, it was only helpful as a sounding board or to give encouragement—mostly about stress in a person's life—not as guide or a monitor for weight loss. This is a very important part of the long-term success, but should not be seen as outside help used to control, manage, or even cheerlead. Rather, it should be viewed as a part of a facilitation that comes with a healthful lifestyle, leaving the responsibility, value judgement, and decisions regarding weight apart from the relationship.

It should be noted that exercise gets double, sometimes triple, duty. As a calorie burner, emotional adjustment factor, and entertainment, exercise plays a vital role. Remember, a weight problem is not an intellectual problem. Weight problems have more to do with emotional matters and how a person handles them.

Factors Important to Enhanced Self-Esteem: High Self-Esteem Brings Self-Efficacy

Members of the 5-Plus Club were questioned about such things as direction in life, change, meaning and purpose, beliefs, and value priorities to see if these factors influenced their ability to be successful. Of course, only subjective answers about these important matters basic to personal development were possible. Still, approximately half of the participants felt they were aware of a strong purpose and meaning in their lives; they stated they had a clear consciousness of their basic beliefs and their top 25 value priorities. If their assessment was correct, they are an exceptional group in more ways than just weight loss. Most individuals I have counseled over the years need a good deal of prompting before they can come up with a clear, extended clarification of their own beliefs and values.

Change—the Key to Success

The last item from the collected data deals with change, particularly self-initiated/self-directed change. Going from chronic weight problems to healthful lifestyles involves a good deal of risk. Twenty-five (83.3 percent) of this special group indicated that they are people who seek out personal change, while 13.3 percent tend to avoid change, and 3.3 percent (1 participant) vacillate.

Desiring and seeking personal change may be the single most important factor in the achievement of success within this group. How each person goes about making changes (whether or not they are in an emotional struggle), and how well they continue to do as time goes by, varies a great deal. It is unlikely that any of these people would be in this special 5-Plus Club if they did not have the courage to face the risks of self-directed change.

145

SUMMARY OF THE RESULTS:
A PROFILE FOR SUCCESS

As stated previously, weight problems have no single cause and probably no single cure. Each person still must deal with a variety of factors that may contribute to their problem and need to be modified in order to resolve the problem. It is obvious within the 5-Plus Club that a great many differences exist, even though all group members have lost at least 20 or more pounds and kept it off for five or more years. If we examine only the half of the group that achieved their ideal weight, kept it all off for over five years, and who were not constantly struggling with themselves to eat and exercise in a healthful manner, we see there are still a great many differences in the ways they have achieved their adjustments. The profile that follows is meant only to give the most common characteristics of one group of relatively successful people. The reader will do well to evaluate this information in relation to his or her own life, viewing none of it as being the perfect answer. In fact, if there is a single answer, it may be that each person has to discover his or her own way.

An example of the caution being suggested pertains to the time taken by each person to lose his or her weight. Every person started with different weight and build combinations; different ages and eating habits; different living and working arrangements; different personalities; different genes and conditioning; different parents, socio-economic status, etc. Some people lost the weight in a few weeks. For others, it took a few years. Even if the mean (average time) is six months, or the mode (most frequent time) is one year, it doesn't take into account all of the readers' personal variables. The time factor was best measured by looking at the pounds lost per week which, for most, was one to three pounds—clearly a much slower rate than most overweight people want it to be.

In other words, most of these participants lost their weight gradually. It is also true that the people who lost the weight quickly tend to be in the group that is still involved in the struggle mentioned earlier. So, even through exceptions always exist, it appears as if learning to be patient and losing weight gradually provides a better chance for long-term success.

New data from studies looking at those who have kept their extra pounds off for five years or more should be out in the next year or two.

If the reader has already developed patience, trying to match the average would not be important. Instead, what would be important is finding what works for long-term success by looking at all the variables, with "gradual" as the guideline.

The following profile is not set up in a hierarchy of priority. The factors that seem to be most common and the most successful will be noted, as will the successful exceptions. In other words, simply remember that regardless of how common each of the factors being considered are to the 5-Plus Club members, it is still extremely important that each person evaluate them in their individual context. Other important variables that are not mentioned here may be revelealed when and if a larger study is done involving different participants.

When you read the following profile, consider the factors as they relate to previous weight loss efforts that you have made and what might fit the situation that currently exists.

A high percentage of the 5-Plus Club:

- *Forego outside assistance,* other than emotional support from friends, spouse, or parents. In the few exceptions where assistance was utilized, it appeared to have been counterproductive. As long as the quest for external magic goes on, then complete, comfortable weight balance seems to be elusive.

- *Obtain emotional release and support* from two or more sources. Exercise and friends were most common sources, as were lots of hugs and regular, satisfying sexual release.

- *Have emotionally stable homes and friends* that function within a healthful lifestyle of self-development, and are able to lend support in a natural way that does not control or attempt to assume responsibility for the overweight person.

- *Have given up smoking, alcohol or drugs* prior to weight reduction, which provided some additional confidence for change as a less stressful first step.

147

- *Have established regular exercise routines* which provided multiple benefits beyond calorie burning and usually were retained easier than other aspects of lifestyle change. Note that participation in sports activities was more of a source for entertainment than it was for exercise.

- *Eat low fat or vegetarian diets for health* rather than for weight loss. Most members of the 5-Plus Club did not count calories.

- *Are involved in on-going education* which, whether general or specific to nutrition and exercise, and whether formal or self-taught, seemed to help them to meet their needs and goals in ways undefined here.

- *Have modified perfectionist traits and rebellious streaks* leading to a more comfortable, less precarious balanced weight. These people were less vulnerable to emotional distress.

- *Are primarily motivated by vanity and health* to balance weight. Vanity was the primary incentive at the start of weight loss, while health served best for endurance.

- *Experience a high degree of career satisfaction.* This seemed to be common to most, together with other major aspects of life (i.e., relationships). Pressure at work was acceptable if the job satisfaction was high.

- *Are socially outgoing,* i.e., comfortable with new people and new social situations. However, being comfortable and "doing it" can be two quite different things. A desire and an active willingness to learn to be comfortable is all that is required.

- *Have reduced the amount of structure and allowed for more spontaneity* in their efforts to change. Finding harmony rather than control is the difference between comfortable weight balance and the struggle with weight decisions.

- *Seek quality in life today and self-directed change for tomorrow* rather than avoid change. Being able to confront their fears of change which had put limitations on their life was a common characteristic of those who were successful.

Realizing self-efficacy may be the most significant piece to the puzzle of why some people's efforts at long-term weight loss succeed, while others' do not. Supplying people with information only when they have a self-determined need for the information they desire and seek may be helpful. Setting up structured programs that smack of control and paying others to take the weight off or to bring about change to them seems to backfire. Information regarding motivation, procrastination, and self-sabotaging behaviors seems to have value only if the weight loss efforts are self-directed. If a person is not seeking self-change but only pursues external magic to change himself or herself, then he or she will not use the information.

WEIGHT LOSS MYTHS

Just as the data I collected accentuate some of the shared characteristics of those who have successfully lost weight over the long term, they also knock down, or at least call into question, some of the popular myths our society holds regarding who can not successfully lose weight. These myths should be challenged.

Myth: Victims of child abuse have difficulty losing weight.

My experience and studies show that between 25 to 30 percent of overweight people have been abused emotionally, physically, sexually, or verbally. Because of this, it is often assumed that those who have been abused will have much more difficulty in achieving their desired weight and maintaining it. Looking at the 5-Plus Club, I found that the percentage who were abused—16 percent—is approximately half that found in groups who have used commercial weight loss programs without success.

Although this may indicate that while having been abused as a child does inhibit assertive self-change efforts, once the efforts are made, the history of abuse does not preclude the possibility of overcoming compulsive behavior over an extended period of time.

Myth: Thyroid/metabolic conditions impede successful weight loss.

Thirty percent of my research group had been diagnosed as having metabolic or thyroid conditions. All but one had long since (prior to the study) stopped taking any medication and wondered whether the medical diagnosis of a thyroid or metabolic disorder had been correct.

In her studies with overweight people using the only reliable measurement of metabolism known to date, Dr. Sharon Alger of the National Institutes of Health found no individuals who could not lose weight on a normal caloric intake. The findings match those of additional medical research undertaken in other parts of the country.

Even when physical conditions inhibit weight loss, they rarely eliminate the possibility. Even those scientists who first developed the set point theory acknowledged that appropriate exercise can change the set point, or metabolic block. In fact, recent research has actually shown that the set point theory is not valid. Within my research group, heart disorders, water retention, and the use of steroid drugs for asthma were all conditions that inhibited weight loss—in addition to thyroid problems. All of these disorders, however, were corrected with lifestyle changes.

Myth: Childhood obesity means lifelong weight problems.

Although the onset of obesity was highest (43.3 percent) during the teen years, especially around puberty, 33.3 percent of the 5-Plus Club members developed weight problems during their childhood and 23.3 percent developed their problems as adults. Sufficient percentages from each group indicate that no matter when weight problems first occurred, long-term weight loss is still possible. In other words, these findings may indicate that poor family eating habits or the development of such conditions as excessive fat cells or slower metabolic rates resulting from age need not determine whether or not a person remains obese.

The percentages pertaining to the onset of obesity are approximately the same in all groupings within my survey of subjects. Those who tried weight programs in the past but dropped out of them, those who lost weight for the first time, and those who lost weight in the past but then regained it were equally successful after five years.

Myth: Poor nutrition and exercise information keeps people heavy.

Even prior to this research study, it was clear that the lack of information about nutrition and exercise was rarely a factor in cases of excessive weight gain. Apart from taking special classes or training in nutrition or exercise, basic information in these areas is and has been broadly available through the media, schools, hospitals, workshops, books, etc., for at least the past 25 years.

The vast majority of clients I have seen in weight loss programs have been exposed to more than enough information about these vital subjects. They know what is fattening and what is not, or at worst, they know how to avail themselves of the information. In fact, people with weight problems tend to be drawn to information about nutrition and exercise. If anything, they would almost have to go out of their way to *avoid* information about these subjects to remain ignorant about the basics of what is and what is not fattening. Although some people may not know what carbohydrates are, if given a choice between lemon juice and mayonnaise, they are easily able to chose the less fattening of the two.

It is also clear that a high percentage of overweight people are very intelligent and well educated. Often they are health professionals such as nurses, doctors, or even dieticians. Nutrition and exercise information is, of course, very valuable for those who wish to use it. Among members of the successful weight loss group, if this type of information was not readily available, the individuals sought it out on their own without any prompting.

Myth: A family history of obesity cannot be overcome in the long term.

Among the 5-Plus Club, 59.2 percent had overweight mothers, while 33.3 percent described their fathers as obese. There was a total of 70.3 percent of the research subjects who had one or more overweight parent. Findings such as these raise serious questions about nature, nurture, family, and cultural conditioning issues as they relate to obesity. Only 29.6 percent of the subjects in the study came from families where neither the father nor the mother was overweight, yet all of the subjects were able to lose weight and maintain the loss. Only 11.1 percent of the spouses of subjects in the study were overweight, which again raises the question of environmental influences.

In May of 1991, the U.S. Department of Agriculture announced the findings of research leader Dr. Paul Moe which indicates no meaningful difference in people's efficiency in food metabolism. This finding supports that of similar research by the National Institutes of Health. This means our genes and basic metabolism cannot be blamed for weight problems. If a person is fifty pounds overweight, they probably have eaten enough to support being fifty pounds overweight. However, exercise is the factor that can change metabolism as well as increased muscle mass which requires more calories to support.

It should also be pointed out that the high percentage of females (67.5 percent) in the research group challenges the claim that because females are more apt to be overweight due to nature's plan, they can't keep it off.

Myth: Depression is tied to obesity and disappears with the weight.

Over half of the members of the research group had suffered bouts of non-clinical depression while they were overweight. After keeping the weight off for five years or more, 20 percent of those who suffered from depression remained depressed to the same degree as they had been before their weight loss, while 10 percent of them were somewhat less depressed, leaving a total of 34.4 percent of the group that remained depressed to some degree many years after losing weight. This represents a 32.2 percent overall decrease in the number of people who experienced depression, but it does raise questions about the role of depression in the onset of obesity and in the loss of excess weight.

Myth: Overeating is a result of liking food.

While there is no doubt that overweight people enjoy the pleasure of food, part of that pleasure is undoubtedly derived from the sensualness of eating. Biochemical comfort results from eating. It is, therefore, not surprising that prior to their weight loss, 70 percent of the individuals in the research group were eating in response to their emotions. On the average, of commercial program participants who regain weight or drop out of their program prior to completion, over 90 percent have indicated that they are "emotional eaters."

Myth: Giving up smoking or drinking is more difficult than losing weight.

Of the 78 percent of the research group who used either alcohol or tobacco, only 6.5 percent indicated they continued to drink socially after having maintained their weight loss for five or more years, and only 6.6 percent of them continued smoking. None of the subjects were ever considered to be alcoholic. Only three (13.3 percent) of this group came from families with an alcoholic parent, and one married an alcoholic. All of those who gave up smoking or drinking felt it was much easier than changing their eating behaviors.

Myth: The chronically obese must have help to lose weight and keep it off.

Seventy-eight percent of the members in the research group had used a variety of weight loss methods— *unsuccessfully*—prior to their last effort, which did prove to be successful. With their last, successful effort, *85 percent did not rely on outside help of any kind.* The remaining few who did continue to use outside assistance did not attribute their success to the to the outside help, but viewed it as a channel for their own efforts.

Myth: Once a person has fallen victim to the "yo-yo syndrome" he or she will never be able to lose weight or keep it off.

In my study, 43.3 percent had "yo-yo'd" at least two or more times prior to their successful weight loss effort. In each case of fluctuating weight, outside help had been involved. All of the group were able to maintain a steady weight loss and keep the weight off when making their final, solitary effort.

Even though a person's metabolism may slow with repeated fluctuations in weight, at least among this group, no one who had previously been involved in weight yo-yoing was prevented from reaching their goal or maintaining it. Dr. Sharon Alger's studies for the National Institutes of Health support these findings. It appears that even if the alteration in metabolism has taken place, it doesn't preclude weight loss or maintenance on a normal food intake. The type of calories eaten, i.e. percentage of fat, may, however, make a difference.

Myth: The more weight loss programs you have participated in, the less chance for success.

Of this group, 76.7 percent had attempted more than one weight loss program prior to their final successful effort. Most of the remaining group who sought help prior to their final effort had used weight loss products, a medical doctor, or some type of therapist or exercise spa. There appears to be no number of prior attempts that would prevent a chronically overweight person from achieving long-term success.

Myth: Counting calories is important to long-term success.

Only two (6.7 percent) of the members of my research group found counting calories useful in losing weight or keeping it off. This means that 93.3 percent of these successful people either found counting calories unnecessary or counterproductive to reaching their goals.

Counting calories seemed to be a symbol of control against which people routinely rebelled. It is my observation that calorie counting also distracts people from becoming aware of the nutritional value of foods and lowers their reliance on themselves to lose weight. Calorie counting can also makes them feel dependent, handicapped, and out of control, as well as exacerbates the tendency to lose faith in their own abilities to find harmony between their emotions and their bodies' needs. Credit for any success tended to be given to whoever set up the calorie count for them, instead of to themselves.

Knowing and *believing* the truth about these myths may change pessimistic attitudes into optimistic efforts to overcome, individually, what commercial programs, medical doctors, and some weight loss groups promote as a "disease" or condition that cannot be "cured" without outside help. Although this small study is hardly conclusive, the numbers are strong enough to indicate that losing extra pounds without help may offer better odds for success than paying for assistance from professional weight loss "experts." It further indicates that larger long-term studies should be conducted to learn if utilization of weight loss programs is counter-productive to permanent weight balance.

Evidence collected by independent sources indicates that individuals succeed in losing weight on their own when they have not been successful using popular programs. Furthermore, commercial or outside help may actually be detrimental to long-term body weight balance.

Instead, by looking exclusively at individuals who have been successful in reducing and keeping their weight balanced for five or more years, it may be possible to verify whether most of them did it by themselves, and whether the commercial programs were either of no help or were even harmful. If these observations are true, identifying the commonalities peculiar to those who were successful might be useful to others who have not yet realized their goal.

Chapter 10

HOW TO LOSE WEIGHT
(NOT MONEY)

*P*rior to entering my *Weight Loss through Wellness program four* years ago, Louise had tried packaged foods, diet pills, aerobic dance, fitness spas, radical diets (including fasting), nutrition classes, twelve-step programs, support groups, hypnosis, psychics, dieticians, and she was even considering surgery. Two years after entering the wellness program, she still had not lost any meaningful amount of weight. During those first two years, Louise continued in the wellness program, joined several other weight loss programs at the same time, read several books on other methods, and took cooking classes. She also bought a treadmill and came to individual counseling sessions.

The extent of her efforts in finding the "magic" solution seemed to be unlimited. Louise always presented herself as happy and good natured. She joked about her search and would acknowledge that "it" (the wellness program) wasn't making the weight come off. In fact, we joked about "it" being "her," not the program. The one thing that was different about the wellness program I offered was that she hung with it, while she would stay with other programs only a short time.

PRINCIPLES OF WELLNESS

The Weight Loss through Wellness program Louise was introduced to focused on a great deal more than what the bathroom scale said. It was focused on true wellness.

Wellness is much more than the absence of illness. It is more than a static state which you attain and then sit back. It is not something another person can "do to you" through treatment or by applying a "guaranteed method."

Instead, wellness is:

- An ever-expanding experience of purposeful, enjoyable living—an experience which you create and direct.

- It is a choice; a decision you make to move toward optimal health.

- Wellness is a way of life, a lifestyle you design in order to achieve your highest potential for well being.

- It is also a balanced channeling of energy—energy that is received from the environment, transformed within you, and returned to affect the world around you.

- Wellness is a process—a developing awareness that there is no end point, but that health and happiness are possible in each moment, here and now.

- Wellness is the integration of body, mind and spirit—the appreciation that everything you do, think, feel and believe has an impact on your state of health.

- Wellness is multi-demensional, and its components include nutrition, physical/emotional awareness, stress reduction, spiritual/philosophical beliefs, and self-responsibility. It is recognizing that the only thing that is certain in the universe is change.

- Finally, wellness is the loving acceptance of yourself.

Humans function as a whole unit and all parts influence all other parts. Therefore, it is ineffective to isolate and adjust any one aspect without considering the rest of the whole. Any program must consider the whole person. The Weight Loss through Wellness program I developed integrated wellness concepts into its consulting services. It considers the environment in which individuals live and work, for they often have a major influence on health factors.

Wellness is an integrated, holistic treatment, but also, and more importantly, it is the prevention of illness and the development of optimal health and human potential. The fact is, human potential is unlimited, and in the process of seeking it we automatically rid ourselves of most ills—plus we can derive new and previously unknown benefits.

LOUISE'S DISCOVERY

A couple things may have contributed to Louise's endurance with the wellness program. She found an intimacy in the small groups and enjoyed the openness and social aspects of it. She relished being loved by the group, especially since she didn't feel loved at home, and there were no great demands or expectations for her to perform in any way.

At the start of her third year in the program, Louise injured her back. It was the result of weakened back muscles and inappropriate lifting. Her pain was chronic and eventually increased to the point where an operation seemed like the only possible solution. She avoided the risk and pain of the operation as long as she could, but with her job on the line, she finally accepted what she thought would be the least difficult of all the procedures. Unfortunately, not only did the operation fail to relieve her pain, the pain became so severe for a time that she was confined to bed and heavily medicated. She was, of course, depressed and added on a good deal more weight.

Eventually, Louise returned to group meetings, painful as it was for her to sit for two hours, and also attended physical therapy for a number of weeks. She improved enough so that the doctor said she could return to work half-time. Louise is now able to tolerate four hours of activity and sitting and is learning to deal with the pain to the point where she can concentrate.

It has been during this recovery period that I noticed the greatest change in Louise. What was just intellectual understanding for Louise before, now seemed to be applied.

Louise's changes also corresponded with her switch from a mildly structured group which was moderately expensive, to an unstructured experimental group with no fee. Louise and I both attribute her change and new found success to the doing without structure or payment for help.

Louise's unfortunate back injury helped her to realize that if she was ever going to improve her situation, it would be the result of her own efforts. Doctors had done what they could, and still she had her back pain. Doctors were certainly even less able to improve her behavior. Also, Louise realized that when she paid for help she quit trying to help herself, and no group or individual counseling session was going to change that reality. When she didn't buy help, Louise was confronted with her own freedom to choose.

In the new group, the people cared, but it was her pain, physically and emotionally. Louise could use the group as a resource, but only she could make things better. Since Louise has developed new insights and made decisions based on them, she has lost a steady one-to-two pounds each week. It may be sad that it is such a slow, difficult process to finally realize what was intellectually understood much earlier, but the kind of change the average overweight person seeks is quick and easy—and does not last. The learning process takes time, but it is what works best.

Understanding change is not enough—we must want to earn it. No, each person does not have to be injured to acquire the changes that last but, unfortunately, that's the way a great many of us come to really understand. Intentionally or not, through their quick-and-easy promises, the billion-dollar weight loss industry promotes the postponement of meaningful, intrinsic change—changes that, when carried out, would result in healthful weight ratios.

Commercial weight loss programs would not comprise the billion-dollar business they do if they were not responding to what is often a psychosocially learned problem and blind demands to have the problem fixed quickly and easily, and with little effort. The skillful deliberateness of the borderline fraudulent exploitation of the vulnerable public needs to be confronted. It is clear that most all commercial weight loss products, programs, surgeries, and services are exacerbating a national health problem physically, psychologically, and economically. It is hoped that these providers of weight loss services will one day be required to inform potential consumers of their failure rates and health dangers.

PAVING THE ROAD TO HELL WITH GOOD INTENTIONS

It is not with pride that I recognize my own part in contributing to the great American fat rip-offs. Coming from a family that had a history of obesity problems and being sensitive to people with this problem, it was always my intention to help. But, in my drive to do that, at times I served the weight loss industry better than those who used it.

Aversion

I first became involved by designing and conducting research for a corporate-owned hospital that was already involved in the treatment of alcoholism and smoking. One method of therapy this hospital used was called "aversion conditioning." As long as it was included in the experimental groups, I was free to try other methods that were safe and potentially effective.

Aversion conditioning deals mainly with the pairing of a negative experience (physical, non-harmful pain) with an old pleasurable experience (eating fattening foods) to create an aversion in the subconscious mind to the formerly pleasurable experience. Once the research design was set up and operational, it quickly became apparent to me that the aversion conditioning did not work. Aversion conditioning, on its own, was the least effective of all the different experimental methods I tried.

I did, however, learn a great deal from using it. First, I saw the power of offering what appeared to be "magic." A small, two-paragraph announcement mentioning my research and my need for subjects in a small, suburban newspaper resulted in over 500 phone calls the first week! The phone continued to ring throughout the next year, just from that single announcement, through word of mouth, and the attention the media occasionally gave to the research project.

When I interviewed candidates for the research, I would try to warn them of the unknown outcomes and limitations in order to keep their expectations down, but it was clear that most of what I said fell upon deaf ears. The people were so intent on being hooked up to that magic box—the quick, easy solution—that they usually didn't even ask about any possible dangers of the program. To them, it seemed that "it" would "make them change," so their attitude was, "let's get on with it." The focus on the "magic" was so great that, until they got what they came for, it was useless to try to talk about other possibilities. Quick fixes are only starting to lose ground today.

Secondly, I learned that once those in the aversion conditioning group realized the magic was far less powerful than their desire to eat inappropriately, they were ready to consider more conventional methods, such as gradual self-change.

Third, the corporation informed me that the high cost of their treatments was a large part of why clients quit smoking or drinking, at least in the short run. At the time and for a long while after, I assumed the corporation's theory was correct and that it would apply to the weight loss program as well. Only recently, when reviewing long-term success rates for all commercial programs, has it come out that paying for help may actually *reduce* a person's chance for long-term success. Experimental group members who are not charged a fee often do better (although not great) in terms of long-term success than those who pay for commercial programs today. Today, preliminary studies indicates that the more people pay for help, the higher the expectations for the program or service to change them, and the less they seek intrinsic change.

Another thing I learned from the aversion conditioning groups was that when the conditioning was paired with imagery exercises (mental pictures), changes lasted longer (although they were still temporary). When I used imagery by itself, I realized it was even more powerful than the aversion conditioning. People who develop their own imagery skills realize their power and confidence to make free-choice changes.

The research also pointed out that a support group's value faded in three or four months. First, I thought that just switching to another group was the answer. I still believed that the longer a person was in group therapy, the better his or her chances for lasting change. Now I've realized that switching groups is what many do to renew the initial value of a group. Like Louise, they keep finding new groups in which to start over. Later, I realized that different people change at different rates, and some actually use group therapy to avoid change.

Of all the different experimental methods I tried, aversion conditioning was the least effective, although a few people would succeed over the long term, even with this method. The two methods that were most effective (temporarily useful) were the comprehensive wellness group and the existential discussion group. The focus in these groups was not on weight loss, but rather on how healthy the member's life style was. Volunteers were not excited about the wellness group, as it was slow and was focused on health, when most of the people in the project indicated that their primary motivation for weight loss was vanity.

The existential group (Freedom to Choose Group), which focused on acknowledging ownership of oneself, including one's thoughts, emotions and behaviors, did as well or better than all the groups, yet they had no "therapy" other than the group. This should have been my biggest clue that expensive, full-service programs will never be effective for large numbers of people. The more that people look to others for change in their own behavior, the less they seek change within themselves. The group discussed why it is impossible to escape our freedom to choose when we are aware of choices. No discussions were about weight loss, diet, exercise, imagery, hypnosis, or anything about their purpose in being there. In fact, other than weighing in to see if they qualified, and weighing at the end of the experimental group meetings, nothing could be construed as treatment for the purpose of weight loss. Most likely, the success of those in the existential group came from their own decisions that any real change was up to them. This group was followed for only a year, but at that point, they exceeded the results of all other groups, except the wellness group. Both these methods would be very hard to market.

The decision by the corporation as to which program to promote was based solely on the marketability of the program, which included the profit margin, and had nothing to do with long-term effectiveness. Because the corporate management knew that aversion conditioning was the least effective, it is hard to believe they didn't also realize it had a limited market life. If my belief is correct, the corporation knowingly marketed a program that was sure to fail in order to obtain the quick profits, or else they believed they could somehow force it to work. At any rate, after my research, aversion conditioning for weight loss was dropped from their treatment programs.

After my experience with aversion conditioning, I ran my own wellness weight loss programs both in and out of the hospital setting. The same comprehensive Weight Loss through Wellness program sold much better in a hospital setting, probably because the average person is conditioned to believe without questioning that "doctor knows best," and that hospitals are where you go when you are sick. Although the wellness weight loss program sold better in the hospital setting, a sensible, no-magic, slow, comprehensive weight loss program will never make the hospital large profits, so it was never promoted by the hospital.

Gastroplasty

During the eight-year period I was running my own programs at one hospital, I was involved briefly with another hospital close by that was doing gastroplasty (i.e., stomach stapling) and liposuction (the surgical removal of fat cells). The patients were having post-operative difficulties. I was asked to take part in their programs because they had no trained counselors, which they had advertised as being part of their program offerings.

After going through the formalities to obtain the credentials required to be on the consulting medical staff and after watching a few operations, I was told I could work with the patients on an individual counseling basis and run weekly group meetings. However, the hospital informed me I could only see the patients *after* the operation. It was quickly apparent that the surgeons did not want me to talk anybody out of surgery for social and or emotional reasons. After I met with a few patients in their rooms and wrote my findings on their hospital charts, the chief surgeon told me directly he did not want me to make any entries in the patient files that would indicate emotional disturbances existed. Two group sessions convinced me that some patients were not only seriously disturbed, but also very angry, feeling the hospital had given them misinformation and/or had failed to give them all the information they needed to be fully prepared prior to signing up for the operation, not to mention the $15,000 dollars they had paid for their unhappiness. The patients were disappointed, embarrassed, hurt, frightened and depressed.

Apart from the promised counseling that had not been provided, the patients had also not been told that their desire to eat would be just as great as ever after the surgery. They had not been told that the vast majority of them would regain all their initial weight loss plus more, and that their stapled stomach could be gradually stretched to accommodate larger amounts of food. Neither had they been forewarned about the pain and discomfort from the foot-long incision or about how many times they would regurgitate their food. Nor were they told they could have many of the same nutritional problems as a person on a partial fast.

Although the numbers reported by marketing people to prospective clients differed, one staff member at the hospital who was bothered by what she saw told me that only 25 percent of the stapled patients retained their initial weight loss after eighteen months. Imagine the statistics after three to five years! In a few weeks, it was very clear to me how totally unprepared these stapled patients were to deal with their rapid weight loss, and how, at best, the medical and administrative staff had mislead these vulnerable people. Even some of the morbidly obese patients for whom the gastroplasty seemed justified because their lives were in jeopardy questioned whether the procedure had been appropriate. They wondered: if they were healthy enough to survive the operation, then weren't they also fit enough for less radical, more gradual weight loss methods?

It is my belief that gastroplasty is rarely, if ever, justified. My experience with the stapling procedure and with stapled patients who have regained their weight and then enter yet another radical program such as fasting, has lead me to believe these individuals were at best mislead by medical literature, medical doctors, hospital administrators, and the medical associations accrediting them. At worst, the procedure is useless and even dangerous, and all those knowledgeably associated with it are insensitive, calculating mercenaries who fraudulently represent themselves, the procedure and its potentials. Why more malpractice suits haven't been brought can only be due to the embarrassment of those who bought into the procedure.

Liquid Fast

After this experience, I felt sure I would never be involved with such abusive treatments again. However, the worst was yet to come. Time, complacency, and frustration weakened my resolve. Giving my attention more completely to my own hospital-based Weight Loss through Wellness program, I encountered a series of frustrations. Hospital administrators would come and go, each one having his or her own ideas about weight loss. But the one concern they all had with my program was, "does the program pay for itself and make a profit?" The program barely did either. It was a program that had no magic. The people who liked it best were those who, through their own trial and error, had figured out that the magical solution they had sought was an illusion, and they were ready to try something new. Also, professionals who had worked with weight problems appreciated the comprehensiveness of the program.

The administrators counted the numbers and quickly became indifferent to the program, to the extent that only if the program did not get in the way of other, more profitable activities, would it be continued. Next to smoking cigarettes, excess weight is the second greatest self-imposed cause of premature death. It would always shock me to realize, once again, that the hospital would show little or no interest in finding healthful solutions and would even support potentially harmful and ineffective methods of weight loss for money alone.

Although my books, magazine articles, and radio talk show appearances would always spark some interest, it was clear that the "quick fix" was in, and if a weight loss program did not offer one, it was highly unlikely to be profitable—with or without promotion. I am hopeful that this situation is changing, and the wise consumer is starting to show greater interest in healthful methods and programs for weight loss.

One administrator told me that because the price we charged was modest, no real profit could be made. Furthermore, if we raised the price, we would lose all the customers. With each new administrator, I would submit new proposals to do more self-funded research as a marketing tool, to assure numbers, gain community recognition, and to learn more about what happened to our clients after the program —not to mention to learn about new and better methods of facilitating weight loss efforts. Oftentimes no response to the proposal would be given, or the administrators determined that my plan was not feasible because it was somehow going to cost the hospital money, even if the project was self-funded. Most of the research literature described biological studies seeking medically treatable problems who could be treated with medication or surgery. My belief was that people remained overweight primarily because of psycho/social causes, and we needed to resolve those if we were to bring change with real, live people.

As I was about to give up on hospital-based programs, it appeared that the situation was going to improve. A new, young administrator was put in charge of my department and indicated she wanted to develop a large, thriving program that would be effective. After all of my years of struggles, what she was saying sounded very good to me. She felt my Weight Loss through Wellness program was excellent but would take too long and be too costly to generate large-scale interest. She wanted to offer a nationally-known program that could be put into place quickly. She asked me to be a part of the search, saying I could still use my expertise at the hospital and do research, also.

It seemed too good to be true, and it never entered my head that anything other than a healthy program would be considered. We looked at several programs which seemed to be both healthful and profitable; however, the program that was finally selected by the administrator met only the hospital's needs for profit. Of course, it was a well-known program which promised big money for the hospital and rapid weight loss for the participants!

I was shocked and argued against it. The administrator called me in and asked if I could live with her decision, pointing out that we could now offer the clients the best of two worlds—they would have the quick fix they wanted, and with my unrestricted behavioral program, they could truly learn how to keep it off, so we wouldn't really be doing any harm. In addition, I could keep my own program, and once the new program brought in some revenue, they would even promote my old wellness program.

Dismayed with past frustrations and lured with the promise of research to come later, not to mention my satisfied ego and an increase to my modest income, I was able to rationalize and justify one of the worst weight loss methods of all, in my opinion: a liquid fasting program. This was something I had spoken out against many times in the past, and I would again in the future.

I told the administrator that I would live with it as long as I was only involved with the behavioral part of the program, and if I would always be free to speak what I believed to be the truth about the fasting program. Such radical programs will usually die of their own weight due to their extremely poor long-term success rate; however, those individuals who are determined to have the "quick-fix" may attempt it a second and third time, blaming themselves before they decide the system does not work. I believed, incorrectly, that the clients would come to that realization at least as soon as those in the aversion program had. However, fasting did provide the apparent results through quick water and lean muscle tissue loss, so the patients reached that conclusion more slowly.

No springboard to change came about. The overweight administrator believed, as did the misguided clients, that *weight* was the block to motivation and change. It was also foolishly believed that because the hospital charged $3,000, it would improve success rates. Instead, what really happened was that participant's expectations of the program and product increased.

The fasting program started about the time Oprah Winfrey made her first announcement that she had lost 67 pounds on a liquid fast. Business was overwhelming. For the first year we were always behind the demand. I hired the best counselors I could get who would work for the low wages and poor conditions the hospital offered. The counselors all held master's degrees, but none had any real experience with weight loss. Their in-service training was hit-or-miss at best, and did not make up for the years of experience needed to really understand the extent of the problem with those people who came in large numbers for a quick fix. These counselors were to make up for what the magic powder couldn't do.

Only one of the medical doctors involved in the program was given a few days orientation to the fasting procedure. He was made the medical director and passed on his "expertise" to several other physicians who wanted to moonlight for easy extra money. All of these doctors worked a few hours each week and none had a background in bariatrics (management of obesity and related conditions), with nutrition or, specifically, with fasting.

The dieticians were already part of the hospital staff and this extra service was added to their regular duties. From private conversations with them, it was clear to me that fasting was not something they believed to be in the best interest of the "patients." They all were young, came from conventional schools of home economics and, like the doctors, had little experience working in commercial programs with large numbers of obese outpatients. Given the position they held, the backgrounds they came from, and their mild-mannered personalities, they were as compliant as you would expect them to be.

Part-time nurses were used as pivotal monitors of "patient" charts, and were delegated the chores of weighing, measuring, taking blood pressure, and setting up for the brief minutes during which "patients" would see the doctors. Together with the receptionist/cashier/secretary, the nurses would dole out the "magic" liquid fasting powder each week. Like the dieticians, they were used to being subservient to the medical doctors and were very unlikely to challenge questionable practices in the program. Two of the nurses in this particular program were also overweight and were participants in the program. They were chosen for this program not because of special training or background with weight problems, nutrition or commercial weight loss programs, but in part because they could serve as role models for the clients/"patients." Interestingly, both of these obese nurses lost large amounts of weight and learned a great deal about the behavior of people choosing rapid weight loss, and yet they fell into the very same patterns of behavior themselves. Even with the insight, support, and motivation/pressure of their position within the program, both nurses were soon on their way back up the weight scale. Becoming disenchanted with the program, depressed, a little angry and embarrassed, they resigned.

Exercise physiologists were also employed part-time to teach basic information about exercise in half-hour segments at several points during the first three months of each person's weight loss effort. Here, too, the physiologists were moonlighting from their full-time position in athletic medicine/physical therapy. These support professionals were also without relevant experience, and at best provided useful information to people who were still focused on the quick program as a source for change.

The front line personnel were part-time college students who assisted one of the only two full-time employees and who together acted as the receptionist/cashier/secretary. In addition to handling most of the paperwork and coordinating with the staff, these people were able to have the most intimate contact with all the client/"patient" complaints and compliments and got to know the clients from a public relations position. They were often the ones in whom the client confided, while professionals were thought of more as authority figures who monitored their successes or failures.

In other words, this set up created an *us vs. them* situation, rather than an intimate forum for change. The client/"patient" could better identify with these young office women who, like them, were directed by those "authority figures."

The next tier of individuals involved in the program was the administrative management personnel. This consisted of the hospital's president, a senior and mid-level manager, and a junior manager. Also, there was a sales representative for the pharmaceutical company franchising the fasting product. With the exception of the senior manager, the hospital people had no first-hand knowledge of the weight loss business or any of the component specialties.

This all added up to a large group of interdisciplinary professionals, only myself having had any real appropriate background with weight problems. Except for two, all of the workers were part-time and were managed by two sales people and a senior manager who was charged with improving the bottom line of the hospital.

To the emotionally-driven overweight person seeking a quick fix, this hospital team and the commercial product touted by Oprah could look mighty impressive. It all made it easy to overlook how this team was put together and what their backgrounds and motivations were, not to mention a client's odds for short- or long-term success.

In retrospect, this program was without a doubt the worst I had ever been involved with, if for no other reason than that its ineffectiveness was well disguised by its professional cover and what appeared to be its comprehensiveness. At least non-hospital commercial programs, products and self-help groups have no real guise of professionalism. When challenged by skeptics, the hospital's defense was to mention the behavioral program they offered with the fasting. In reality, behavioral methods have been shown to be only slightly longer lasting than other methods of treatment for weight loss. Between the fact that the program was known to be ineffective, and that it was adopted by the very pharmaceutical company which sold its materials to the hospital administrators, odds for success were slim at best.

Behavioral methods vary a great deal, and the quality cannot be standardized any more than those who use it. Even if one behavioral method or counselor may have better methods than another, no research can repeatedly demonstrate long-term effectiveness.

Starting as we did with an overwhelming number of clients, eager to buy into another dream, a basically untrained and part-time staff, the powerful money motive driving the hospital management, and no proven methods or means of weight loss to promote, it was a miracle we had as few problems as we did. Because these radical programs are ineffective and are popular for only a short time, they still continue to rip off the emotionally vulnerable of millions of dollars.

In hindsight, it is easy to see why radical programs like fasting, aversion conditioning, and stomach stapling should be regulated. Even at the time, I knew we were taking in people who had no business being in such a program. We knowingly accepted individuals who were in bad physical shape, who were alcoholic, elderly, lonely, clearly unable to afford the program, and who were emotionally unstable and unable to functionally utilize the program. At the time, my protests were often weak, rationalized, and unspoken. "Strike while the iron is hot" was the motto and we kept it all moving along. We put our heads in the sand and put the little bit of extra money in our pockets, and my guilt grew with each passing day.

In time, just keeping busy was not enough to keep me distracted. Gradually, it became very clear that the business profits were not being used to build a solid, long-term, well researched, healthful program. After every request to do research or to promote the Weight Loss through Wellness program was unanswered or denied, the mid-level manager finally told me the program would be ended as soon as it was no longer profitable.

The terms "client" and "patient" being used together is one example of how the whole philosophy of hospital-based programs makes it unlikely that long-term change will occur. To be a "patient" is to have a medical problem and to seek or receive medical care. The word "patient" describes someone who is ill or injured and who must passively wait for recovery. Although some of the individuals who took part in the fasting program had maladies that might have benefited from medical treatment, for most of these "patients," fat wasn't one of those maladies. Fat, in and of itself, is only a potential precursor to illness.

By calling the clients "patients," the professional staff and the pharmaceutical company implied that a medical treatment is available to cure fat. The patient need only be passively compliant and, *voila,* the fat will be gone—he or she will be "cured." Long-term change requires a proactive client who fully accepts his or her power in a situation that is basically one of free choice. At best, those who facilitate the process are only supportive educators.

The whole program was a setup for the Great American Fat Rip-off, an expensive facade of comprehensiveness, run by professionals, in a trusted hospital setting. Underneath, it was loosely coordinated, it utilized poorly trained professionals, was pushed by a sales-oriented pharmaceutical company, was run by a hospital in financial difficulty, and was under the supervision of managers whose jobs rested on the quarterly bottom line. Add to this an overweight population living in a society obsessed by the compulsion to meet acceptable standards of thinness—most of whom are perfectionists with $3,000 worth of expectations, low self-esteem and fear of rejection—and you have a formula for a very popular and profitable fat rip-off.

To make the point of what a powerful role emotion plays in this whole scenario, it should also be noted how broad the spectrum of consumers is. Rich and poor, young and old, black and white and everyone in between seems to be attracted to the illusions of magic. There were not only uninformed people buying into the magic illusions but also professionals of every kind. Medical doctors, counselors, nurses, engineers, CPA's, teachers, business executives, lawyers—all of them bright, well-educated people with access to the information they needed to make sound, logical decisions not to enter programs of this type—would join with the less informed, sharing the belief that if they could just get the weight off one more time, they would keep it off for sure, discounting any self-image changes other than the physical. Believing that the fat somehow kept them from changing on their own, they thought that once the fat was gone, they would be in "control."

CREATING A PROFITABLE ADDICTION

I have mentioned only those programs which I believe to be some of the bigger rip-offs, with which I have had first-hand experience, and which were run in a hospital setting. Many, many other commercial programs exist, each getting their share of what is reported to be a $100 billion dollar pot. Some of the people who run these programs are well-intentioned, but most are contributing far more to this national health problem than to its resolution.

The obesity research files are full of sound studies that are truly objective and a great many additional studies that may look objective but were funded by the companies that sell the weight loss products and are not identified as paid research. Taking into account the likelihood of biased research, I have yet to find one study that shows, without a doubt, that any product, treatment, theory, or service has been repeatedly effective in the long term (5 years and more) for more than 5 percent of the subjects studied.

Much has been learned about how people deal with weight behaviorally and psychologically. We know that people do change, they can lose weight and keep it off for long periods of time—even a life-time. My own follow-up study of the 5-Plus Club members and the research of Dr. Schachter of Columbia University analyzes those people who have been effective in keeping the weight off for a long period of time.

In his book, *Diseasing of America* (Lexington Books, 1989), Stanton Peele, Ph.D., fully disputes the belief that people who drink too much, eat too much, or spend too much do so because they have an illness. Such a belief is absurd, he asserts. Dr. Peele claims, "the disease theory of alcoholism and addiction is an elaborate defense mechanism that evades the real issues we face as individuals, families, communities, and as a nation." These real issues deal with questions of existential choice and self-awareness. Dr. Peele feels that providing people with a "lifelong disease" sets them up for relapse and retards their personal growth. It is his belief that we are conditioned to fear our environment and to believe we are out of control in it.

As a means of escaping our fear and regaining control, we turn to compulsive behaviors and then label our compulsions a biological disease for which we don't have to be responsible. The treatments for these "diseases" become our new dependencies, be they medications or lifelong therapy groups. He points out that, if excess weight were primarily a genetic or biological problem, we would not have a 54 percent increase in obesity among children ages 5 to 11, or a 98 percent increase in the prevalence of the morbidly obese in this same group since the mid-1960's.

We have more fitness centers and exercise facilities and larger numbers of people using them than ever in the past, but the percentage of people getting heavier keeps increasing. The more treatment programs and doctors working in them, the more weight problems we have. By creating a disease diagnosis, we shift the emphasis from social and cultural to individual causes and cures, creating a boom in the weight loss business.

Dr. Peele seems to be saying: first the world sets up a condition of social distrust and fear from which we isolate ourselves into our homes and out of the community. The media, news and entertainment reinforces the fear, then advertisements and doctors convince us we are helpless to deal with our emotions and condition (disease) alone, and we buy into a system that not only doesn't solve the problem but makes it worse.

He also brings a great deal more documentation to the idea that compulsively addicted people do much better with their own efforts than they do by being helped within the medical model or through highly structured self-help groups or commercial programs.

WHY MILLIONS PAY BILLIONS

Stories like Louise's abound. Radical treatments, such as those I have described in this chapter, have been failing for decades (see Preface), and the libraries are full of independent research indicating that programs and products don't work. Professionals like Dr. Peele and myself have written books on why treatment for compulsive behaviors don't work, and how they damage the chances for possible success. Even Congress has supported what former Surgeon General C. Everett Koop pointed out: i.e., that "quick fix" weight loss does not bring long-term success. Furthermore, it is also known that:

- The body has a higher percentage of fat each time lost weight is regained

- The yo-yo syndrome leads to a metabolic condition that allows the body to stay overweight on normal amounts of food

- Each time a higher weight is achieved, additional fat cells are permanently added

- Weight loss diets are most often diuretic diets and nutritionally unsound, leaving the dieter more vulnerable to illness

- Weight loss diets often get rid of more lean muscle tissue and water than fat

- Weight loss diets are most often boring, bland, complicated, inconvenient, tasteless, strange, or costly, and cannot be continued for a lifetime

- Dieters seldom stick with a weight loss diet long enough or consistently enough to lose meaningful amounts of fat, and if they do, they are in danger of harming themselves physically

- After the rapid weight loss diet is over, it leads to a greater volume of food eaten or greater cravings for fattening food

- Each time the weight is regained, the next weight loss effort is more difficult, both physically and psychologically

- Many deaths, illnesses, and emergency operations have been linked to quick weight loss methods
- The quality of medical care offered in weight loss programs is most often low
- Large amounts of money paid to providers of services, treatments, and products are clearly the main motivator for the fat industry
- FDA warning labels are required on many weight loss products
- Low calorie diets shut the metabolism, thyroid, and sympathetic nervous system down to low gear, depriving nonessential body functions of energy, causing short-term symptoms (i.e., loss of hair) and long-term damage to other organs
- Rapid weight loss leads to the body's over-production of the enzyme lipoprotein lipase, making it easier to put the weight back on.

This is all public knowledge and easy to tap into, so why do such commercial programs continue to draw large numbers of hopeful clients/patients into still more fat rip-offs? We now know of the many outside forces at play and the power they bring to bear on the continued growth of the nation's girth and the oftentimes damaging, mostly valueless, use of products, programs, services, methods and techniques by the hundreds, while millions of dollars are spent annually doing research for the next magic bullet which will be heralded as the forthcoming panacea to do it all for us.

If we do not look at what isn't working or why, with our history of conditioning to believe it can't be done alone, how much interest do you think exists for even examining those who do have personal long-term success? Are people interested in the psychological understanding and personal insight of why they fail to develop the patience, take the time or the risks, or make the changes gradually?

The effort, time, desire, belief, and hope to do the more difficult things that will work have not been emphasized enough to pull the overweight person's attention away from magic bullets. The pressure of overwhelming change, the necessity to have two incomes per family to stay afloat, endless competition, a distrustful world offering little caring, and high expectations for fat-free-foods and pills that burn fat during sleep, also make any realistic, relaxed focus very difficult to sustain.

Showing interest in bottom-line factors, such as overcoming perfectionism and low self-esteem; developing true healthful eating patterns; and conquering fears and self-doubt while learning to change taste preferences can seem like too much for one person to take on alone, so why not go one more round, trying to beat the odds? Achieving long-term success through a fat rip-off may be expensive in many ways and have very poor odds for success, but to most people, doing it alone seems even less likely!

Yet, there are signs that the numbers of people finding the inner harmony on their own is growing. We are starting to look at those who have made it, instead of only those who do not. The scientists and corporations who believe compulsive people cannot do it alone may be put out of business one day in the same way the tobacco companies in this country are threatened by an informed public and increased regulation and advertising constraints.

Once enough individuals start to believe in and understand themselves, and get mad enough to say, "I won't buy it anymore!" the whole national problem may turn around rather quickly. The profiles in Chapter 9 describe individuals who have found their harmony and weight balance long-term. Try to realize *they* are the models for you, and that you can be the model for someone else.

Chapter 11

WEIGHT LOSS GROUPS
Helpful or Harmful?

*L*ouise had been in one weight loss group or another for approximately ten years. Some of the groups she attended were as small as three or four members, and others as large as forty or fifty. A few of the groups were more like a class where the "leader" was teaching something, with limited input from the members; while other groups were open discussions of topics decided by the members, and the "facilitator" stepped in only when the group was stuck. Most of the groups in which Louise participated were task-oriented and had clear goals and objectives, while others had a continuing theme but little structure. One group had no structure other than the stated intention of each group member to actively work on self-identified changes.

The many leaders and facilitators of the groups in which Louise had taken part were as different from one another as were the personalities of each of the composite groups. Education levels, credentials, experience, attitudes, personality traits, income status, emotional stability, professional backgrounds, philosophical orientations (e.g., religious to parapsychological), age, and gender were all variable characteristics of leaders and members.

Some groups were very conservative; others were very liberal. Some groups stuck rigidly to topics such as diet and exercise, and others talked about any and all subjects. Some groups were very tightly bonded and the members were faithful to one another and their group leaders, while other groups had a very rapid turnover, and few friendships were developed. A number of times Louise felt frightened when powerful emotions were expressed and horrifying stories were told, or when group members would get into a confrontation that couldn't seem to be resolved. If nothing else, Louise was knowledgeable about groups; she knew the role she would play in them and how to manipulate each group session away from her hidden concerns.

For Louise, group had served various needs, including: entertainment; an escape from a house without love; a social network to develop friends; a place to play and laugh; a distraction from her pain; and a place to hide from her concerns while receiving emotional support and positive confirmation. The only thing Louise really didn't like about group were the times a group leader or facilitator would bring the group's attention to bear on her and ask serious, confrontational questions about her feelings and thoughts.

All in all, Louise felt support groups to be positive. They fulfilled many of her needs on a short-term basis. The question was, did the groups serve the purpose for which they were designed, i.e., in any way did personal growth or meaningful change result from the many hours and money spent in groups? Was Louise any better off for having attended them, or did the group only provide an entertaining opportunity for further procrastination? No permanent weight loss was apparent; therefore, were other benefits overlooked?

The answers to these questions may be very subjective and difficult to assess; however, after examining both the intended purposes of the group and Louise's stated intention, a few conclusions were quite clear. When Louise finally stopped being part of a group, she was functioning at a higher level of self-efficacy than at any time during or prior to attending groups. Judging solely by her statements and her appearance, it seems as if she is now more consistent with her diet, exercise, personal growth (assertiveness) and relaxation program (tai chi) now, without the group, than she ever was in the past.

Louise believes she acquired more than enough information to deal with diet and exercise, long before she made any real effort to use that information. She now feels that the unrestricted, unstructured groups gave her the most insight into herself and to helping her understand why she wasn't using the information available to her. However, she still cannot understand why she continues to procrastinate. She acknowledged using the groups for all the wrong reasons mentioned above and feeling guilty at times for knowingly doing so without admitting it to others or, at times, even to herself. When the last group ended, she knew she didn't want to seek another, and she felt a little lost and panicky about just what to do. She also felt sad and a little depressed, as though she had lost a good friend. Louise knew she could contact any of her old group members, but she also knew it would just be another way to procrastinate. She was frightened, but she didn't want to go back or to hide any longer from things like fattening foods. She wanted to change her people-pleasing, caretaker, co-dependent non-assertive behaviors. She just wasn't sure how to bring the changes about.

Then the tai chi experience came along, and things were very different. Louise had not belonged to any sort of group for several weeks. She did not feel as though she was looking for a substitute for group. She had more or less let go of her weight struggle when she noticed the tai chi class in the park. Louise does not believe she was drawn to tai chi for any of the old reasons which had formerly drawn her to all those group sessions. She had no role to play out in tai chi as she had in other groups. She had no ulterior motive for attending these classes. She was not even there for weight loss reasons. She was there to experience the movement. Except on the occasions when her teacher asked her to help with a demonstration, she did not feel that she was "performing" for anyone. Her experience with tai chi wasn't like her aerobic weight loss classes either, as neither she nor anybody else had any expectations for anything in particular to happen as a result of the class.

Very little talking was done with other class members or by the teacher—it was mostly just practicing the movements over and over again. With the practice came the calm yet energetic feelings. Her moods improved, she felt better physically, her little nervous tics started to disappear, and her back even felt better. Her interest in and attitudes toward food were changing to the point where she noticed it—but she did not get all excited about gradually losing a few pounds. Her focus stayed on the movement and the satisfaction she felt with the practice.

The second time her teacher asked her to help with a demonstration, Louise realized that she had changed herself. Louise felt alive and more certain about what she could do. She felt she was in harmony with herself and her world; and what fears remained, she knew she could deal with. Although she knew life wasn't perfect, and may never be, she was still okay.

It is true Louise was still part of a group (class), but now she was in a very different group. She used the group simply as a means of channeling her efforts. She no longer focused on outcomes or social approval. She had allowed herself to look inside without intending to do so. Very little of what went on in class was intellectual or even verbal, and yet her insights and understandings about herself seem to be realized in a way they never had been before. Louise was empowering herself through *mastery* which made her wellness lifestyle information easy to use. She didn't go into the process with the intention of gaining harmony; it came as a by-product of the practice.

In my book *Change Your Mind: Change Your Weight*, (Health Plus Publishers, Sherwood, WA), the chapter "Putting It All Together" includes a section on support groups. Those pages still seem to be as true today as they were in 1985, the year the book was published. They discuss how to select a group, how to get the most out of group, the way group is intended to function, how to assess the leader, your opportunity and responsibility to benefit from group, etc. However, something is missing, and that is what *this* chapter is about. My earlier book does not explain how and why groups can work against you. Nor does it offer a clear explanation of what, in my opinion, is the most important aspect of group: *proactive change.*

The group "leader" is the take-charge person who determines the direction and topics, who instructs group members on how to correct their concerns, and provides organization (structure). Usually, he or she will not risk confronting individuals for fear of being seen as unkind. A group leader will modestly accept praise (credit) for group or individual success and perceived personal growth or short-term weight loss, and overlook weight that is regained.

In very subtle ways, possibly even unnoticed by the group leader, the supportiveness of the group results in a bonding of the people who are a part of it—which the leader is apt to take credit for—and gradually the group becomes dependent upon itself. Individuals who feel that they cannot continue their short-term success on their own are often fearful of loosing the group, and they may turn to the group to "save" them. The "leader," blinded by his or her own ego needs, revels in the flattery and tries to assume the protective parental role and "rescue" the members who are still full of self-doubt, possibly after months or even years of attending group.

No individual is really at fault when this happens, not even the group leader. The group dependency comes about as a result of co-dependent personalities who gather together with their caretaker/people-pleasing skills in full force, liking one another for that reason, sharing and laughing in a way they usually don't at home or work, and having a leader who needs approval and praise as much as anyone in the group does. Analyzing their concerns and seeking answers with the group and "leader" quickly seems comfortable. Receiving praise and approval from the group for small changes, and comforting reassurance for slips in their organized plan, makes the usual self-critical self-talk go away for awhile. The co-dependent group becomes like an extended family and members are able to hang onto each other for a while.

Even if this co-dependent group extends itself far beyond the scheduled time, things usually start falling apart within six months or so. Many of the participants who don't lose much weight early in the program drop out. Others who have lost weight start to regain it and are embarrassed to return to group. A smaller number of hard-core members will stay with the "leader"—many times for years—and add or continue individual counseling with the "leader," having faith and rationalizing improvements in an almost neurotic/symbiotic relationship. Popularity, new dependencies, avoiding discomfort, entertainment, extended families, on-going psychoanalysis 101, and "guruitis" were never what anybody intended the group to provide. It happens because individual group members and the group as a whole are avoiding risk, challenge, or fear, or the program is being perpetuated for financial reasons or possibly for the leader's ego needs.

Although most groups are well intended, some have less than altruistic motivations. If the sales pitch is based on following the rules, i.e., eating "their" packaged foods, relying on fasting supplements, or taking shots, etc., then, as a rule, the group or program includes simple, infantilizing (you're not bright enough to figure it out yourself) behavioral methods which are stressed over and over. In these cases, the overweight person is relieved of the responsibility of making decisions, learning to believe in himself or herself, and taking responsibility for the long-term outcome. Short-term credit always goes to the product, service, or guru ("leader"). When the weight is regained, however, blame is placed upon the group member for not staying with the rules.

A true group "facilitator" would not be hawking products, books, programs, or extended packaged services. The "facilitator" will be very clear about his or her limitations, and will not encourage prolonged group attendance or a continual review of old theory or personal problems and treatments. Nor would the facilitator set himself or herself up as the centerpiece to bond to, the final word of wisdom. Almost everything the facilitator does should be aimed at helping the members need the group less by finding the answers they need inside, or achieving self-efficacy (a belief in the individual's ability to change himself or herself). Group would not be focused on the personal problems of one member for long periods of time, while the other group members sat quietly, un-involved. Credit for short-term achievements would be given to the individual, and they would be given minimal attention compared to change of the underlying causes affecting long-term outcome. The facilitator is more like another group member who sets up an environment that is conducive to self-directed change.

In other words, group can be an instrument of change, or it can be a means of avoiding change, or it can become another form of dependency.

GROUP CHANGE

Group is intended to assist each member's efforts toward self-directed change based on new self-awareness, emotional ownership, a greater sense of confidence so that members can risk making change, and a place for each member to realize the self-efficacy that allows for adjustments to new life contingencies. Toward this end, group intends to:

- Nurture each member's abilities and sense of strength to be able to function on his or her own beyond co-dependency/caretaking

- Encourage adaptation to new circumstances

- Assist in redirecting external focus on the approval, direction, expectations, motivation, and strength of others to each member's greater appreciation and understanding of his or her own beliefs, values, worth, and intrinsic drives to be what he or she chooses to be

- Provide a sense of community, new information, a forum to express individual opinions and receive feedback, a supportive sharing that can lead to insights, and opportunity for personal development apart from the group

- Facilitate individual choices to change with optional means and methods (e.g., letting go of critical self-talk and replacing it with affirmations), and

- Aid in adapting to new circumstances, people and places.

There are primarily two types of group that are ideally suited to achieve the above-defined purposes of a group and each member's personal goals. One type of group has to do with *self-understanding*. This type of group is designed to serve as a diagnostic self-exploration dealing mostly with how individuals in the group came to be the way they are, why they feel about themselves as they do, why they behave as they do, and why they hold the values they have. In addition, it helps members to determine what changes each person would benefit from by making; and which of those possible improvements they are "willing" to work on. Basic characteristics of this type of group are:

- Small, e.g., comprised of eight to twelve members

- Clarification of group process is provided by the facilitator

- Open to an examination of all relevant subjects

- Involves discussion (expression and feedback) of personal thoughts and feelings

- Eclectic verbal methods are taught by facilitator, such as role play, and

- Emotional support is verbalized and confrontation encouraged.

The second type of group is the *proactive* group. This group is meant to go beyond analysis and emotional support. The proactive group is for individuals who already believe they have a good grasp on who they are, how they came to be who they are, what they want to change and what they are willing to work on changing. The basic characteristics of this group are:

- Stimulation and support of gradual, self-determined developmental activities (change through risk-taking);

- The use of identified concerns (fears) to strengthen self-image through social, physical, intellectual challenges;

- Discussing and planning appropriate challenges for members;

- Discussing successes or difficulties from attempted challenges and possible adjustments for future efforts;

- Attempting first challenges within the group;

- Defining new personal social, mental, physical potentials through discussion and spontaneous activities created in group.

This proactive group is meant to bring about the changes that diagnosis, discussion, and support rarely do, for it encourages action. *Action* is necessary to bring about change of our beliefs about ourselves. When we see ourselves repeatedly doing something we have avoided in the past, doing those type of things becomes easier each time, the threat goes away, and our confidence grows.

AN EXAMPLE OF A PROACTIVE GROUP

The intention and purpose of a proactive group is to stimulate and support gradual, self-initiated personal development activities (change through risk-taking). A proactive group is ideally a vehicle in which each group member uses his or her own fears, questions, and problems to strengthen his or her self-image through the use of intellectual, social, and physical challenges. The objective is not only personal change that is wellness-oriented and holistic, i.e., covering body, mind and beliefs, but also change that results in the discovery of new, self-enhancing potentials.

Proactive group sessions may include:

- Defining personal fears, questions, and problems

- Discussing/designing appropriate challenges for group members, and

- Analyzing challenges, reviewing the successes, making adjustment and planning second efforts.

The "menu" of challenges supplied on later pages presents three levels of difficulty. The individual can proceed through these levels gradually, at his or her own pace. In the first series, the challenges are completed in the group setting. The challenges in the second series are completed outside of the group but together with one or more supportive individuals. The last and most difficult series includes challenges to be completed by each member on his or her own. This menu of challenges can be modified or adapted to individual needs or used as a basis for creative efforts by the group members to design and plan their own.

The degree of risk encountered in each activity is determined by the group member. What may be difficult for one member may be very easy for another member. The idea is to always be in a process of identifying, planning, confronting, relating, or adjusting challenges to be faced, advancing to more difficult challenges as the member's confidence grows. Keeping activities frequent will speed up ever-developing self-esteem. Any challenge that is resolved will improve a person's ability to deal with matters of choice, such as diet and exercise.

To be fearful is an opportunity to know your courage. Because every activity is self-initiated, honest and open sharing is essential for personal success. Only the individual can know for sure how much of a risk he or she is taking, but even other people who know the risk-taker may notice changes in self-esteem, image, trust, confidence, and belief if the individual has taken true risks.

CHALLENGES

Proactive risk-taking is not done for entertainment or thrills. It is meant to be done with serious intent, planning, and care. The purpose is to improve one's self-image, self-trust, and self-confidence.

The main fears common to all humans are:

- Fear of pain (physical/emotional)

- Fear of embarrassment

- Fear of losing what we have

- Fear of not getting what we want, and

- Fear of fear.

If we listen to our bodies (which will express our emotions to us), then we will know when we are out of our comfort zone and close to our fears. Once we become aware of discomfort (fear), the risk is in confronting it.

THE "MENU" OF CHALLENGES

Series I

The following challenges (i.e., risks) are meant to be done within the group setting. Each group member chooses and/or designs his or her own challenge, selects the time to confront it, and determines whether it will be done alone or with other group members. Consider these challenges to be a warm-up.

1. Lead the group in a self-improvement exercise, using details from a group exercise guide or a self-created plan.

2. Do a reading or act out a scene that takes you out of the character type people know you by.

3. Sing a song that expresses some strong feelings either to the group or one individual in the group.

4. Give a serious, prepared ten-minute talk that supports an idea you are very much against.

5. Tell two group members what you believe would make them more successful and popular.

6. Do a dance that tells your story of fears and hopes.

7. Do five minutes of stand-up comedy.

8. Express yourself for three minutes without protecting your self-image in any way (i.e., be fully yourself).

9. Communicate your feelings non-verbally to another group member or to the full group for five minutes.

10. Share a creative idea or poem you've written with the group.

Series II

The following challenges (risks) are meant to be done outside of the group setting with another group member or person of your choice. All aspects of the proactive group will still apply. You are in charge of knowing when you are out of your comfort zone or if you should withdraw to prepare for a later attempt. It is not necessary to put your personal safety in jeopardy to achieve your goal. Just getting on stage makes you a success.

The following menu of suggested activities is offered only to stimulate your own imagination. You can pick from the menu if you like, modify something from the menu, or create something special for you. Keep in mind that allowing time for careful planning is one thing, and procrastination is another.

1. Work a day at a food for the homeless dinning hall.

2. Go for a small plane ride or take an introductory flying lesson.

3. Conduct a survey at the airport with of at least 20 people.

4. Caddy for strangers at a golf course.

5. Put on a *bring-one-person-you'd-like-to-meet* party. (Each person from a core group of friends brings a new person that other core members don't know but are apt to enjoy

meeting. Thus, everybody at the party gets the chance to meet new people.)

6. Put on a new games party for families, with no food.

7. Climb to a peak that is higher than you've ever been.

8. Apply for a job for which you have no experience.

9. Ride the city bus as far as you can on a single ticket.

10. Create a healthful (non-fattening) dish and try to have it put on the menu of a local cafe.

11. Make a dramatic change from the hairstyle you currently have.

12. Develop a dramatically different clothing outfit that is a departure from your usual style of dress, and wear it.

Series III

The following challenges are meant to be done by each member independently. All aspects of the proactive group still apply. You are still in charge of knowing when you are out of your comfort zone and if you should withdraw to prepare for another attempt. If your personal safety is in jeopardy, your first priority is to reevaluate your path to your goals and take a less precarious road. You are still able to pick from the "menu," modify a "menu choice," or create your own challenge to fit your needs. Remember, the closer together you experience challenges, the sooner the changed view of yourself will come about. You are the boss!

1. Describe your philosophy of life, and compose your value priorities list (see Chapter 5).

2. Spend a full day relating to people without using your voice.

3. Spend a Sunday visiting with the elderly in a nursing home.

4. Make a gift and give it to a person you care about when it isn't a special occasion.

5. Spend a day in stores, offices, and cafés and meet at least eight people. Find out what they are afraid of.

6. Meet with authorities from religion, art, law, and education and ask: "why can't people get along with each other?"

7. Put yourself in situations where you tend to be impatient, and while you wait, figure out why you are so impatient.

8. Spend a weekend alone in a hotel, camping, or any place you can be without books, radio, TV, or other distractions.

9. Arrange to ride in a police car for several hours one evening.

10. Arrange to do cold-call selling for one full day.

Monitoring your own feelings and setting up your own challenges will undoubtedly serve you the best. A proactive group that is used well will serve as an initial base and a means of channeling your efforts, as well as a launching pad for future efforts on your own. If you find yourself in a group where you are no longer acquiring new insights and where you are not initiating your own new efforts, it is very possible you are in group for the wrong reasons.

Group support is not for everybody with a weight problem. If the individuals in the group are not growing beyond the need for the group, the group may be more beneficial to those who set it up than it is to the members. Whatever the group is, remember "it" is not going to change you—*you* are going to change you. Self-change is the change that lasts. If you have reason to believe you could benefit from group participation, consider all types before you decide which group is right for you. Depending on your situation, a toastmasters club or tennis club may be more valuable to you than is therapy or a proactive group.

Last but not least, try to gather some statistics on the long-term benefits of any group you are considering. Determine the philosophy, personality, intention, and needs of the group "leader" or facilitator. If you can clearly see within a few weeks that you are not making good use of a group, then it is probably time for re-evaluation or departure.

Chapter 12

WISE CHOICES
ON-THE-GO

Labels, Cafés, and Travel

*L*ike the rest of modern America, Louise was always in a hurry. If she wasn't working, going to a meeting or to the doctor's office, she was exercising, taking a class, or doing something with a friend. As was often the case, Louise would make exceptions to her commitment to eat a healthful diet and make a temporary switch in value priorities. She would momentarily overlook her resolve to eat a healthful diet in order to keep up with her busy schedule or to avoid keeping others waiting, or because she was just too tired to be bothered with all the details of trying to live a healthful lifestyle. She would do things like skip label reading in the grocery store, go to just any fast food restaurant, or choose whatever was on the menu in order to hurry back to work. On trips out of town, it became a matter of just doing whatever her friends and relatives were doing because everyone was tired or impatient. Of course, on special occasions, such as office retirement parties, birthdays, holidays, a night out with friends, weddings, graduations, etc., the list of reasons to depart from her plan would go on and on. So many exceptions were made, in fact, that the exceptions became the rule. Louise would think to herself, "I've broken my commitment so many times that I may as well just forget about trying to eat in a healthful manner."

It does seem like we have a slim chance in a fat world. "Good intentions are crushed by the circumstances in which we must live our lives," Louise would tell her weight loss group. Louise wasn't that much different than millions of others who blame a lack of time, circumstances, or other people for their not being true to their "diet commitment."

Now, of course, Louise does not use a weight loss diet. Like so many others, she has learned that weight loss diets do not work! Counting calories does not work for most people, and being in a constant struggle over decisions about whether to stay with a healthful lifestyle or give in to emotionally pleasing, fattening pleasures is usually a short detour to gaining the fat back again. Breaking the cycle of weak commitments, counting calories, and internal struggles has to do with changing food taste preferences, learning to be sensitive to messages from your own body, taking chances, letting yourself relax, knowing value priorities, beliefs, and gathering information. This chapter is about the information and adjustment alternatives in those difficult situations away from home and on special occasions.

It will be assumed here that the reader wants to make personal changes, live a healthful lifestyle, and utilize information that will be helpful in achieving these goals. Without a strong desire for personal change and the adoption of a healthful lifestyle, little information about weight loss ever gets used very long.

DECIPHERING LABELS

To make valuable use of the information on labels, some general information about nutrition is required. Learning the information provided in the Chapter 7 on the System for Healthful Eating could be a basic first step. Taking classes on healthful nutrition and cooking, and reading a few books and/or articles on nutrition will, at least, provide the basic information about how to limit the amount of fat, refined sugars, white flours, salt, and excessive protein in your diet.

First, it should be known that the U.S. Food and Drug Administration (FDA) is the primary regulator of food labels. These are voluntary regulations and come from the Federal Food Drug and Cosmetic Act of 1938. Few changes have been made in these regulations since 1973. It should also be known that the purpose of labeling is not only to protect the consumer, but also the seller. Some major food items, such as meat, are not required to have labels at all; others, such as most seafood, are not even inspected. Meat and poultry products are regulated by the U.S. Department of Agriculture (USDA). Finally, the Federal Trade Commission (FTC) regulates claims in food advertisements.

Because of shoppers looking for packaged foods with magic health bullets, profit-driven food marketers, and very inadequate government regulations or enforcement, food labels are not only misleading and confusing, but all too often they are even fraudulent. Attention-getting words such as "no cholesterol" are emblazoned on packages of products that may actually raise your cholesterol level or be laden with other fats. Possibly even worse than what is on labels may be what is omitted from labels.

There are other things, such as chemical additives, fillers, colorings, growth hormones, alcohol, antibiotics, nitrates and nitrites, that are often found in foods and are often considered harmful, or at best unnecessary. Then, of course, there are those things that are found in or on food that are not mentioned on the label at all, like pesticides and rodent droppings. As long as they don't exceed specified amounts, the product still meets government guidelines.

Nutrition labeling appears on the majority of processed foods. Labels will list such things as grams of fat but they provide no information regarding how much fat is too much. And, of course, we don't grow up learning the metric system in this country, but that is how labels list content amounts. Graphics could simplify the understanding of labels using pie charts and symbols with keys.

Terminology

Misleading terms are used, such as "low" cholesterol for which there is no legal definition. It is not explained that tropical oils, such as palm, palm kernel, and coconut and other saturated oils lead to fats in the blood. Cholesterol is found only in foods with animal products, but since you don't know if peanuts are roasted in cottonseed and/or peanut oil, you can only guess whether or not the nuts will have a cholesterol-raising oil in them.

Other terms, such as "high fiber" and "2% milk" are also very misleading. How high is "high," and what kind of fiber is it? How much is enough? One package may contain one-tenth the fiber of another brand of equal size, and still have large red letters touting the fiber content as though it were loaded with it (approximately 25 grams of fiber per day is recommended by some authorities).

Another confusing matter is that the amount of fat in products is given as a ratio to the product's *weight*. What the consumer needs to know is the percentage of fat in the *total calories* of the product. For example, in "2% milk," the fact is that 38 percent of total calories in the milk are derived from fat. If you are interested in limiting your fat to 20 percent or less of your total dietary intake, this kind of information is very important.

On labels, the meaning of words, such as "reduced," "light," and "natural" are also confusing. With sodium, for example, words like "very low sodium," "sodium-free," "salt-free," "no salt added," or "no salt" do not mean the product doesn't contain sodium. The ingredients may contain baking soda or soy sauce, which could raise the sodium count significantly.

The word "light" can mean just about anything from more water, to fewer calories, to a paler color, to a thinner cut, etc. A similar meaningless term is "natural," which also has no legal definition. In addition, the words, "no sugar added" should never be taken at face value. Always read the labels looking for the hidden sodium or sugar, noting what is natural in accordance with your own definition.

Even if a product lists its ingredients in descending order of predominance by weight, it often does not tell the percentages that make up these rankings. If percentages are given, the percentage of calories would present a much different picture to the consumer then the percentage by weight does. Milk is a good example of this difference: 2 percent fat by weight equals 38 percent fat by calories; 1 percent fat by weight is 23 percent fat by calories, and skim or "non-fat" milk can run as high as 16 percent fat by calories. Using deceptive labeling practices such as these makes it difficult for the consumer to realize, for instance, that 50 to 75 percent of calories in ketchup are from sugar or that mayonnaise is usually 100 percent fat. When foods such as ketchup and mayonnaise have actually been improved by replacing vegetable oil, egg yolks or sugar with more healthful ingredients, they can no longer legally use the names ketchup and mayonnaise. In other words, many foods like ketchup, mayonnaise, and macaroni fall into a category called "standardized" foods and can be sold without ingredient lists. Only those ingredients that are classified as "optional," because they are not a part of the official FDA recipe, must be mentioned in an ingredients listing.

Another misleading promotion method is indicating on the wrapper or the advertisement that the contents are "whole grain" or "real fruit." The whole grain or real fruit may be only a small percentage of the total volume. Although by weight the item may be listed first, it may comprise only four percent of the calories in the product. Manufacturers may use similar methods to confuse the reader regarding oils. For example, the words "may contain one or more of the following: olive and/or coconut and/or palm kernel oil." Olive oil has far less saturated oil then the other two, but the consumer would have no way of knowing which oils are actually in the product, and in what ratio.

"Natural flavorings" can mean just about anything with regard to their source or origin. Natural food (i.e., health food) stores tend to sell products that can be trusted to a higher degree in terms of healthful qualities and how clean and environmentally conscious the manufacturers of the products are but, even here, such terms as "natural flavorings" are commonly found, and adequate nutritional labeling is missing about as often as it is in the more traditional food stores.

Placement

The nutritional labels themselves are often hard to see or read because of the size of the print, where the print is located and the type of wrapper on the product (it is difficult to read print on a transparent or shiny, bright, light-reflecting paper). Often the store will put price labels over the nutrition label. In addition, letters are sometimes run too close together, or ambiguous wording may be used.

Sugars

Sugars come in many different forms, and shoppers are confused when manufacturers list it by one of its many different names. Whatever the type or name, it is still sugar and tends to have the same negative effects. Honey, maple syrup, and grain syrups like rice and corn, barley malt, dextrose, sucrose, fructose, brown sugar, and white sugar all need to be considered when the percentage of calories from sugar are counted up. It should also be noted here that artificial sweeteners, such as sorbitol, aspartame (Nutrasweet), etc., by volume, have about the same calorie count as sugar but a higher intensity of sweetness. As it relates to weight loss, people who use artificial sweeteners tend to gain more weight than those who use regular sugar. They conciously or subconsciously believe that "no sugar" means they can afford to eat more calories, and tend to go overboard. Different forms of salt/sodium (e.g., monosodium glutamate "MSG") are also found on labels in terms unfamiliar to the general public.

Chicken

Chicken is yet another concern. When a chicken product has a nutritional label that does not specify "chicken meat" or "skinless," it probably will contain chicken skins. Turkey franks are another good example. Because they are made with the skin of the turkey, the fat content is 71 percent—almost the same as the fat content for beef franks. The use of the skin makes a great deal of difference in the amount of fat in the product. Other products, such as fish fillets and peanut butters can also be vague or misleading regarding their fat content.

Fat

Although most labels include the number of calories per serving, the fat-finding formula when reading labels on packaged foods begins with allocating 9 calories to each gram of fat; therefore, to calculate the percentage of calories derived from fat for any food, multiply the number of grams of fat by 9; then divide by the total calories; then multiply by 100. It is really not even necessary to calculate beyond 9 calories for every gram of fat. Once you know that figure, just by looking at the total calories you can tell if the fat content is too high.

Organic vs. Non-organic

In 1989, spending for food labeled organic increased 68 percent after much national publicity regarding the pesticide scare resulting from the use of alar by apple growers. In most states, however, we have no laws regulating the use of the term "organic." On a national basis, the future for legislation requiring certification standards for organically grown produce and grains looks bright.

There is a struggle over current legislation regarding meat which is called "organic" or "natural." All this should prove helpful to the consumer trying to get away from unwanted pesticides, hormones and antibiotics. However, it can't be depended on, for while some states have laws, others have only voluntary guidelines and are not always monitored.

If you prefer environmentally friendly products, some consumer groups want to introduce product evaluations based upon raw materials and manufacturing, consumer use, recycling, disposal and even genetic alterations. The process will include a review and comment period on proposed product criteria.

Read the Labels

Treat each label as if it were a contract. Read it carefully, do your calculations, look for any tricks in the fine print, write or call the toll-free numbers supplied if the labels are incomplete or unclear, talk to store owners and managers, check in with the Center for Science in the Public Interest (202) 332-9110 and, of course, push state and federal legislators for label reform. The point is, don't trust labels—ask, learn, and eat fresh food whenever possible.

EATING OUT

In the past, when Louise was to dine out with friends and was asked, "where would you like to eat?" she usually answered, "wherever you prefer would be fine with me." Always wanting to please others for fear of rejection, her answer had become a habit she did not have to think about. Gradually, however, Louise has become more assertive (risk-taking) in trying to take care of herself and live closer to her own values. Most of the time these days she will discuss the matter and explain her interests and needs. Sometimes it will take a little longer to decide, or they may drive a little farther, but usually, at worst, a compromise restaurant will be picked. Often, a friend will actually prefer a more healthful meal. As far as I know, Louise has not lost one friend over her new assertive behavior, and she has discovered a few old friends are now easier to be with. She thinks more of herself for sticking more closely to her own values, and her healthful choices are becoming preferred. And, she's losing weight. Louise's friends are also seeing her in a new light of greater respect, which frankly both surprises and pleases Louise.

Finding the appropriate eating establishments has also been a process for Louise and her friends. At first, it was small changes, such as which pizza place had whole wheat crust, requests to go light on the cheese, and selecting vegetable toppings. Then, it progressed to going where there was a salad bar with a really big variety which would sometimes include pasta and Mexican fixings, along with the marshmallow-jello dishes and a fruit bar. The fresh seafood restaurants that would broil the fish were popular for a while and, of course, the oriental cafés that would leave off the MSG and had a variety of vegetable dishes seemed like alternatives which most of her friends would go along with. Over time, Louise's choices have evolved into still more healthful choices. The meat, fat, sugar, and salt in most of her first choices became less and less acceptable. She learned how polluted the fresh seafood from fish farms are and even decided to drop that alternative.

As Louise became more selective, the number of eateries in which she dined as well as the number of times she ate out declined; however, she became more and more satisfied with the restaurants she did frequent. She knew what she wanted in each place and how to order when she would go to cafés that offered few choices that fit into her new standards. Except for a couple of vegetarian restaurants, Louise used standard guidelines as she reviewed the menu offerings in new or less-than-desirable dining choices.

Her first question was always, "May I get side orders that aren't on your menu?" Her second question was, "Will your cook modify servings from your regular fare?" Another solution may be to go to a large chain grocery store. Many of these stores now have salad bars available many hours of the day or small amounts of produce and packaged goods or drinks may be purchased and taken back to the office or car to eat. The grocery store is especially good when traveling by car. Larger food stores usually have a variety of drinks and packaged foods that are kept chilled. Items such as non-fat yogurt, fruit flavored mineral water, whole grain muffins with raisins, and other items are available, and sometimes they even have tables in the store where you can eat. Walking through the grocery store to see how many new ideas or healthful foods you can find can be fun.

Many towns also have natural food cooperative stores. These, of course, are primarily food stores which are owned by the members who also often do much of the work of running the store. Members also vote on the kinds of products the store will carry. These stores have been created not only to provide the most nutritious and clean food available (e.g., organic produce), but also to keep the cost of the food lower by joining with other co-ops to purchase in larger quantities. These stores are usually warm and friendly places which are often more relaxed than traditional supermarkets and they provide good service that will make you want to come back again. The Gentle Strength Co-op, which is located in Tempe, Arizona, close to where I live, also has a deli with booths inside and tables outdoors on the patio. They even offer entertainment on warm summer evenings. The cost of eating there is very reasonable, and it is a place where people can go to escape from the madness of the world. The deli food is simple, nutritious, and tasty. It is also a place where someone with a weight problem can pick up a lot of new ideas on how to prepare non-fattening dishes.

Lower costs, healthful and clean non-fattening foods, and a pleasant, relaxed, friendly atmosphere are characteristics of most co-ops. In addition, co-ops often offer many educational classes dealing with health and the environment at a no charge or a very low cost. Most co-ops are very supportive and active in the community in areas such as helping the homeless, and some are also politically active. It is not necessary to join a co-op or be an active member to shop or eat at there, but you might find that working as a member in such a store can provide other kinds of satisfaction.

Whenever I arrive in city or town on business or pleasure, I check the yellow pages under "health foods" and look for co-ops and health food stores. If I do not find anything listed, I call a health food store close to where I am located and ask them if they know of any cafés, delis or grocery stores where I might find the kinds of healthful foods I am looking for. Usually there is at least one option reasonably close by.

Two less favorable options which I have felt compelled to choose at times are to have a small snack which I pick up at a health food store to tide me over until the next meal, or to simply drink some clean water and miss a meal. If you wish to lose weight and the meal missed is in the evening, no physical harm should result. However, I do not recommend that missing meals become a regular practice, and if you choose to fast for more than a meal or two, I recommend that you only do so under the supervision of a well qualified, experienced health care professional—and never for the purpose of weight loss.

Health food stores, to me, are a mixed blessing. They often are the only place where certain health-oriented products can be found. I believe they do serve a purpose and provide an alternative to the limited choices that have been available in more traditional supermarkets. I also believe health food stores have helped to bring about some long-overdue improvements by major food store chains in the products they sell and the contents of those products. They have helped to put pressure on the medical community to recognize the role of food in the cause and/or prevention of many health problems and as an aid to improving ill states of health. However, health food stores and some of the companies that make health food products still leave much to be desired.

Even in health food stores, it is necessary to read labels, to know what constitutes healthful nutrition, especially according to your own definition. It is important not to count on the store clerk to diagnose or prescribe treatment for any symptoms or special needs you may have. Do not seek magic from any product or jump to the conclusion that the substances you ingest are responsible for what ails you. Many factors influence your state of health and physical fitness, and easy, quick answers which seem too good to be true probably are—especially where weight problems are concerned.

If you shop in health food stores, take the time to get to know the people who own and operate them. Know what you want when you go in and rely more on your own knowledge and that of your health care practitioners (provided they are knowledgeable about nutrition) than on information and opinions given to you by a clerk who has been trained by the company for which he or she works, especially if that person is making a commission on whatever it is they are selling you. It is not my intention to condemn all health food store clerks or owners; some are very knowledgeable and may even have more training in nutrition than your M.D.; however, they are not in business to practice medicine, and you need the best help you can get if you do have a problem. You may need information from a variety of sources, and you are responsible for collecting that information before making your decision about it.

It is my hope that you will check with all your health care practitioners to make sure they have a wellness orientation and that they have a strong academic background and experience about the particular problem with which you are presenting them. This may seem like a major departure from the topic at hand; however, it is also apropppriate and important to take the same degree of responsibility when shopping in health food stores. Ultimately, you are the one asked to take precautions and to assume responsibility, no matter where food your food is purchased or from whom you receive health care advice.

EATING ON THE ROAD

Many of the suggestions mentioned in the previous section are even more appropriate in situations involving traveling. Requesting food choices not offered on the menu, dining in grocery stores, using the yellow pages to find co-ops and health food restaurants, and even skipping a meal are all options that can be useful from time to time, whether you are in your home town or on the road.

When I was a child taking trips with my parents, I remember my mother packing huge lunches that could have fed several children for several days.

Usually all we would purchase would be beverages. My mother did this more for economic than for health reasons, but the idea has served me well on many trips. Bringing your own food takes some planning and increases the amount you will have to carry, but it is a popular alternative for people who travel and are interested in healthful eating. Some major celebrities will not only carry their own food for themselves and their families but also will bring cooking utensils and other equipment, such as blenders, to use in their hotel rooms. Many hotels provide kitchenettes for guests who wish to prepare their own meals. In fact, most of the better hotels and motels have rooms which come with a small refrigerator, sink, cupboards, and some type of small stove or microwave oven.

You can shop at grocery stores, health food stores, and co-ops to stock up either before you leave or when you arrive at your destination. When traveling by car, it is easier to take the perishable food already in your refrigerator, prepare large amounts of hot-plate type dishes, such as vegetable stew, and eat it in the car, as well as in the motel room. Fairly large coolers with artificial ice, packed well, can carry a great deal of food. Regular ice will also work, but it is messier to deal with.

Most of the time when you travel by airplane, the flights are of short enough duration that it is not necessary to eat during the flight. If, however, you are going to eat meals on the plane and you don't wish to bring your own meal with you, when you purchase your ticket arrange to have special meals brought on board for you. Be forewarned that you may not always get the best, but usually it will be adequate. The airlines make a few different types of special meals. I have learned, for example, that just asking for a vegetarian meal does not assure me of healthful food. Either request that no fat or sugar items be included in your meal or inquire what will be served in their different special meal categories on your flight, and you should be able to get something close to what you want. You pay handsomely for your in-flight meals. Most airlines have developed a system to conveniently handle your requests, so that there is no reason to feel guilty about causing the airline any additional trouble.

When you visit relatives and friends or dine out with them, it is certainly considerate to let them know about your food preferences and assure them that they need not go to any special trouble for you. If you stay at their home, do as you would at a hotel and bring as many of your special foods as is reasonable.

Generally speaking, people who like you will enjoy the opportunity to do something special to please you—as long as they don't have to continue doing so on a permanent basis. I have also found that my friends and relatives like to know how and why I eat the way I do; if for no other reason than that they are curious, and a little discussion about it is interesting to them—as long as it doesn't go on too long. Other people have special health or sports needs and are interested in any advice that might be helpful to them, as long as you don't play doctor.

Dining out with business contacts or having a snack at their office during long meetings may pose more of a problem. In this situation, people still want to be helpful and may even discuss it a little, but much less so than in a social situation. This is the situation in which I have most often gone without a meal or snack. If possible, talking with the person who is providing for or ordering the in-office lunch, rather than dealing with your business hosts, is your best chance to get what you want without putting anybody out or taking up pressured business time.

SPECIAL OCCASIONS

Unfortunately, holidays, birthdays, and celebrations of every kind often revolve around food and drink. Because we have a social tradition of believing that we are not having a treat, a "special" good time, or even tasty food unless it we are "treating" ourselves to something unhealthy, it is our attitude and belief about what is "good" or "special" that needs changing, as much or more than the food and drink we consume on these occasions. In some areas of life, special occasions occur all too often. Weddings, promotions, graduations, babies, congratulations, and even divorces and funerals can be just some of the all-too-often special occasions. Any excuse to "fall off the wagon" can be found if you are really looking for one. This is why it is so important to learn to change food choice preferences, not only on the basis of nutritional value but also on the basis of changes in taste preferences and changes in attitude. When you truly believe you prefer the taste of healthful food, and you feel like you're having a treat when you're eating healthful food, then the struggle is over—you need no more advice, and you don't feel cheated or deprived.

When possible, bringing your own food, even for special occasions, is, again, good advice; but be sure to let the hosts know ahead of time. Healthful, low-fat eating has become so commonplace that most good hosts anticipate requests for it and provide something for their health-minded guests. Nevertheless, it is still wise to let them know ahead of time and offer to assist with some ideas, at least, and a food contribution would be even better. Where pot-lucks are concerned, bringing a special dish that is both healthful and tasty will usually go over well. Non-healthful eaters generally get excited about healthful foods when they also find the food tasty, and usually they acknowledge their surprise and pleasure. Often they want to know where they can get this low-fat, healthful food or how to make it. If you choose your dish wisely, I am sure it will be a big hit.

Entertaining or hosting people whom you know to be junk food junkies may be more difficult. I usually warn guests ahead of time and try to offer a wide variety of healthful items. If you provide a number of items, most people will be satisfied with enough of the food to enjoy the occasion. It is very important not to change your own values and priorities. If you want to believe in yourself, it is important to live by your own values and accommodate others within those values. I do not serve my friends and guests food or drink I feel is unhealthful for me to consume. I will go out of my way to try to make it pleasurable and tasty, but I stick with the criteria that it must be healthful. When I have asked clients in my office if they would knowingly serve health damaging food to people they care about, the answer has generally been "no." But, if we look closely at what they usually serve their guests on special occasions, the answer more accurately should have been "yes." When asked that question, they assumed I meant something that would immediately make their guests ill. They didn't think about the slower killers, such as fats, refined sugars and flours, alcohol, etc. Your guests may also enjoy the "new" healthful food because they see the occasion as a nutritional adventure. I have even had friends proudly boast later about the healthful meal they experienced, as though they had just eaten snake for the first time and had lived to tell about their enjoyment of it!

Without adjusting your taste preferences to healthful food, it won't become a priority which you

Without adjusting your taste preferences to healthful food, it won't become a priority which you choose routinely. If you eat healthful food often, without telling yourself "it's not your preferred food," you will come to like it.

Chapter 13

PROCRASTINATION TO MOTIVATION

*W*e are motivated to inaction just as we are motivated to action. If we procrastinate, we most likely have a reason for putting off something we think we want to do, something we should do, or something we have to do in favor of higher motivational drives. One thing I know for sure is that chronic procrastinators are not lazy people. Moralizing and labeling them as lacking ambition or discipline only reinforces their sense of inadequacy and prophesies an expectation they are more apt to live up to. I also do not believe that procrastination is merely due to the lack of organization.

Where consistent, long-term behavior is concerned, such as with weight loss, organization may only add to the problem. Remember that people who are successful in losing weight and keeping it off over the long term and who are comfortable with their behavior achieve their success through spontaneity, rather than through plans, structure, organization or increased "control."

At some point, all humans engage in procrastination. How frequently and regarding how many different matters, varies from person to person. Sometimes we are very much aware of why we procrastinate, sometimes we do not wish to know, and sometimes it is just puzzling to us. Procrastination as it relates to weight loss is one of those puzzling times.

Louise felt she had explored the depths of her soul, and I know for a fact we attempted to explore the depths of her mind, trying to discover why she did not do what she was so certain she wanted to do.

"If you consider the thousands of dollars, the time, and the energy I've spent trying to get the pounds off, isn't that proof that I really want to be thin?" she would say with great emotional pain.

Louise and I considered many possible motives for her procrastination about losing weight. One of the things Louise procrastinated about was making a decision about which of these possible motives was at the core of her procrastination. All the reasons sounded plausible to Louise. For example, if Louise lost her extra weight:

- She wouldn't know for sure if her husband only loved her for her body;

- She would be giving in to her husband's control;

- She would become promiscuous because more men would want her;

- She would no longer have an excuse for facing difficult challenges she was avoiding;

- She would lose attention and sympathy for her unsuccessful attempts;

- She would lose a part of her identity or part of herself;

- She would lose her excuse for falling short of her goals;

- She would lose her power to manipulate family and friends;

- She would lose some of her "friends" because of her success;

- She would have no means of rewarding herself;

- She would lose her means of diminishing anxiety through the comfort of food;

- She would lose her means of achieving pleasure;

- She would lose her means of relieving frustration and feelings of deprivation;

- She would lose her means of expressing hostility;

- She would lose her means of diminishing insecurity;

- She would lose her means of self-punishment to soothe her guilt;

- She would lose her means of proving her inferiority;
- She would find it harder to avoid maturity;
- She would have no means of diminishing her fear of starvation;
- Etc., etc., etc.!

Even if one or all of these motives were true, it could be all it would take for Louise to procrastinate about her weight loss. Yet, Louise always felt that even if all these reasons were true, something still deeper in her subconscious, was really at the root of why she remained overweight. Perhaps at the root of her procrastination was a trauma she had experienced as a child that was too horrible to recall.

What Louise very much wanted to believe was that it was something beyond her control or something she knew nothing about; something that would relieve her of the responsibility to do anything and, most of all, something that would justify her avoiding to take action that she believed would only lead to failure. Without knowing "for sure" what was wrong, avoiding the risk of failure was certainly justified.

Louise, like so many others, was bright and able to rationalize. She was able to create reasons to not follow through with her plans, to find ample cause to avoid her fears, and to look like a martyr, a caring mother, a loyal friend, and a selfless person who always put the needs of others ahead of her own.

Many theorists lean heavily on oral fixations learned in the childhood experience of bonding with their primary security/love object during the feeding experience and to the experience of underfeeding or overfeeding in response to the cries of the child regardless of the hunger need. It does happen that overprotective parents and "busy" parents often use food to deal with all the child's emotional needs, or as a cure for boredom, or to express love. ("Nothin' says lovin' like somethin' from the oven.") As the child develops, the line between physical hunger and emotional needs blurs. Eventually, the overweight person may not recognize hunger pangs at all because all the other stimuli that are responded to by eating seldom leaves time for the hunger need to develop.

For Louise, the blur of possible motivations to eat inappropriately and to stay overweight cleared up as she calmed herself.

By mastering the Chinese movement exercise tai chi, she became more focused and, thus, more calm more often. When we are relaxed, at peace with ourselves, and feel safe, then we see ourselves more clearly and sense our emotions, drives, and intuitions more accurately.

As Louise stayed calm for longer and longer periods of time, her need to eat inappropriately grew less, until true hunger pangs were actually felt again. Because her ability to focus and sense her feelings had improved a great deal, she realized what was happening within herself. Louise also realized that her strongest drive was for affiliation, the need to feel close, loved and accepted by important people in her life.

Because she came to feel more safe in her adult world, she was also able to recall events that had taken place with her father when she was a child and realized it was unlikely that he had sexually molested her, but that he had frightened her so badly on occasion that she had blocked out the memory of those events. Mostly, the fears were regarding possible physical abuse and abandonment threatened by her drunken father. When drunk, he would state these threats so graphically that Louise could not bear the thought of them. By feeling safe in her world today, Louise was able to open the door for these powerful, overwhelming memories to come to the surface of her consciousness.

Some methods for exploring subconscious motives are hypnosis; tests, such as the Thematic Apperception Test (TAT); and psychotherapy. However, the best method is through well-practiced relaxation techniques. The point here is that only Louise could know the answers for sure; the rest was all speculation, analysis, and guess work. Some of that analysis was correct but it was never provable or complete until Louise was ready to re-experience her deeper fears.

Knowing why people hang on to the habits that keep them overweight doesn't necessarily mean the behavior will change, but the new-found certainty of what needs to be dealt with makes denial difficult at best, and procrastination more uncomfortable. Understanding our motives can be very confusing when they are tied into our past experiences, ever-changing circumstances and the emotions that have conditioned our behavior from childhood. A great deal of the process Louise went through to understand herself and avoid her fears was part of the learning process necessary to a full understanding and clear perception of herself. The only qualification was that the whole process of finding her way did not need to take nearly so long. Many of the commercial programs, diets, and gurus had served more as distractions and escapes, without which Louise could have succeeded much faster.

PROCRASTINATION

Chronic procrastination is not just a bad habit but a way of expressing internal conflict and protecting a vulnerable sense of self-esteem. Few people give up procrastinating until they understand the function procrastination serves in their own lives. They also need to know why their self-esteem is low and how putting things off acts as a buffer for their shaky sense of self-worth. Learning to find the energy and courage to get beyond procrastination is, of course, the beginning of changing this defense mechanism that puts too many limits on the potentials of an exciting life.

The Cost of Procrastination

The cost of procrastination for the seriously overweight person is very high. Even though at the time of confrontation of one's fears it may seem easier to avoid the fear, the price paid in the long run is much greater if we procrastinate than it is if we confront our fears. Here are some of the costs of procrastination:

1. *Emotional Pain:* Guilt resulting from knowing what "should" be done, fear of what others will think, and embarrassment when others know. Anxiety, depression, loneliness, obsessive compulsiveness, even suicide may occur in this circle of self-defeating behavior.

2. *Low Self-Esteem:* We tend to believe about ourselves what we see ourselves do. Chronic procrastination leads us to believe we are incapable, undependable, undeserving, inadequate and unlovable.

3. *Lost Opportunities:* Achievement, money, relationships, a sense of aliveness, meaning/purpose, may all slip by the procrastinator,

but, worst of all, the opportunity to like, trust, and believe in one-self is lost by not deciding to take action that works.

4. *Decreased Productivity:* Without action, fewer goals are achieved in most areas of life. The procrastinator then believes he or she is a failure, feels depressed and has little energy to try the next time, which means more procrastination. Logically, of course, putting efforts off and postponing needs always means less gets done.

5. *Troubled Relationships:* Significant others lose respect, trust and confidence in the procrastinator. Procrastinators are often perfec-tionists, and may be critical, easily upset, hurt, disappointed, an-gered and, worst of all, fearful, meaning the "real" person is not seen, making them very difficult to like or get along with.

6. *Impaired Health:* Procrastinators are more easily distressed, and distress leads to illness. Putting off the activities of a healthful lifestyle may mean continued obesity, a weakened heart, high blood fat, more colds and ailments of all kinds, not to mention emotional disorders, such as depression, anxiety, and serious mood disorders.

7. *Loss of Time:* Procrastinating often means wasting life's most pre-cious commodity—the time we have to live—by waiting for con-ditions to improve and for our fears to vanish while we do busy work to distract attention from what is important, and missing fulfillment by living in the past, future, or fantasies. Not being in the "moment" is putting off the opportunities to experience joy, happiness, and enhancing self-worth with a sense of being alive—all of which are found only by living on the edge of our comfort zones.

It is clear that procrastination is not an intellectual matter, but rather an emotional one. The cost of procrastination is too high to be a choice of logic or reason. Bright procrastinators, however, are very able to rationalize and convince themselves that their procrastination makes sense and serves a purpose. We can cleverly tie our postponements into the category of higher values, especially if what we are putting off helps us avoid a fear. We can, for example, be a martyr for our children's needs. Who can point a finger of blame when our reasons for procrastination are for the job (family income), our friends, our spouse, or a parent, and not just a selfish need of our own? Procrastination can help us to avoid confronting our fears of success, guilt and new challenges, but it also can provide us with the rewards or secondary gains of revenge, power, and rebellion to which we may not want to own up.

To find overriding motivations for the reasons we use to justify our procrastination and then rearrange our value priorities, is to realize that motivation builds on itself. To enable ourselves usually takes more than one insight, one event, or one person; it takes a whole series of self-initiated actions done with some regularity, such as the following list of risk-taking tips for letting go of procrastination and beginning to make the changes you need for weight loss.

Letting Go of Procrastination

It is not important that you stick to this entire list of suggestions or that you follow them in any specific order. What is important is that you keep the action going, that you are sincere and realistic with your efforts, and that you are willing to take some risks, knowing that most of your efforts will pay off if you do not overwhelm yourself with your expectations and are willing to get up and try again when you fall down. Choose one or two of these suggestions and give them an open-minded trial. Some will appeal to you, others may not. Choose those which best fit your circumstances.

1. Monitor your self-talk to notice the mental struggles (conflict) going on over what you logically believe (e.g., eat healthy) and what you emotionally want (e.g., to eat fattening foods). Learn how to quiet your mind through the practice of meditation, yoga, or tai chi, and/or learn and practice the basic steps of the "System for Healthful Eating" (see Chapter 7). If you follow through on any of these tips, the mental struggle about what you are choosing to eat will stop.

2. Listen to your body to learn of your fears. Instead of avoiding your fears, gradually and deliberately go toward your fears to desensitize yourself and learn that you are able to resolve them. From this behavior, you learn to trust yourself and reduce your need to procrastinate.

3. Confront your feelings of guilt by practicing "active forgiveness," by taking time usually given to being responsible "for" others and using it being responsible "to" others. This means being a model for others, instead of a servant for others. Set the example of becoming healthy, happy, fulfilled, and of liking the person you are.

4. Stop being critical of others by not blaming yourself for your imperfections. This will take you a long way toward being less angry and thus diminish some of the need to be overweight.

5. Be willing to take some measured risks into the unknown with the awareness that some efforts will not pay off the first, second, or even third try. Both negative and positive risks in changing can be scary. Choose the ones that you can like yourself for taking, even if they don't pay off in the way you had originally intended.

6. Avoid analyzing and judging the meanings and feelings of others— learn to inquire and listen with an open mind; listen without judgement, analysis, or preparing a response, and notice the pay-off.

7. Track your emotions with a daily log of events and your reactions to them. Ask yourself many times each day, "What am I feeling?" and listen to your body for the answers. Notice how increased self-awareness improves your decisions and disposition.

8. Each time you realize you are emotionally upset, ask yourself five times quickly: "What does this mean in relation to my whole life?"

Notice that each suggestion to reduce procrastination requires action and some sort of consistent effort to follow through or change. These suggestions, like any number of others, can be something more to procrastinate about. The difference between these activities and those that have been procrastinated about is only the purpose, otherwise they are identical; therefore, unless you have an extremely strong drive to become a non-procrastinator or have strong motivation to follow these tips for other reasons, it is unlikely the tips will be of great help to you. No matter what action it is or what is being avoided, if the procrastinating behavior is to change, motivation is the key ingredient needed.

MOTIVATION, INSIDE AND OUT

Where does motivation come from? Are we born with it like intelligence; some people with more, some with less? Is it something we learn from our environment? Can we learn to have more of it, especially about important needs we have? The questions can go on and on without any better answers than the tips given above. The answers may be uncertain, but the truth of the matter is that people change from procrastinating to taking action every day, and it seems we all have the ability to do it.

No doubt, if you are over the age of eighteen, you have probably seen yourself stop your procrastination and become a regular doer of at least one thing you had previously avoided. A few examples are:

- Learning to dance even though you think you have two left feet
- Giving up footballs for dresses
- Flossing your teeth daily
- Wearing makeup
- Voting
- Wearing a seat belt
- Organizing your tax papers
- Preparing meals
- Exercising
- Changing an attitude about school, religion, marriage or your parents.

217

Some of the things that you quit putting off you actually learned to like, and some of them you waste great amounts of emotional energy disliking but go right on doing anyway. No matter what it was you stopped postponing and started doing regularly, you created a drive, a reason, a purpose, and a motivation (or many motivations) to get yourself to do it. You wanted something more, you feared something more, you feared something less, you understood a consequence better, you paid the price for procrastinating one too many times, your longing became overwhelming, you hurt too badly physically or emotionally, it was the only socially acceptable thing to do, or you simply came to realize you could change, and it made sense to do so. In any case, there was a possible payoff, benefit, or reward or punishment of some kind that you perceived which helped to bring about the change.

If we do not have enough motivation or motivators to stimulate action, we tend to look for ways to make change easier. The commercial weight loss programs want to appear to be the ticket. The programs, products, or services promise to require less effort (e.g., drive or motivation) from us so we do not have to rearrange our motivation priorities. The motivations to lose weight do not have to be strong enough to override any of the existing fears or rewards. The idea is that we can have our cake and eat it, too.

External motivators (such as commercial weight loss schemes) are an excuse to procrastinate about learning to develop better *intrinsic* motivation skills. Most of us know that changing in order to please family, friends, or a spouse does not result in lasting changes, and even most weight loss programs talk about *doing it for yourself.* It is easy to repeat this statement and believe that you mean it. Yet most of the motivation from any weight loss program is intended to be external. You need to look clearly at just who it is you want to have feel better. Will you put your personal health care ahead of your job requirements, five to ten hours each week? Do you want to live to see your kids grow up so much that you will change the family menu, or make your own healthful meals separately while continuing to fix the usual foods for them?

Chronically overweight people are so used to putting the perceived demands of others ahead of their own needs that it is hard for them to know for sure what is for them and what is for others. It is also hard for this same group to understand just what a motivation to take care of themselves is all about.

When asked the question, "What does doing for yourself mean?" the most common responses are: "it is when I take bubble baths," "buy myself some new clothes" or "do less house work." Seldom is "doing for yourself" seen as action leading to having a healthier mind or body, nor is "making decisions based on personal values and needs" seen as leading to greater self-esteem. Of course, rest and escape activities are useful also, but exactly how is a person going to develop the self-efficacy they are missing by taking a bubble bath? In fact, lazing in a bath only tends to validate one's poor self-image, creates feelings of guilt and promotes a need for more sensual comforting in the form of food.

To chronically overweight people, reaching for external support seems easier and safer than developing self-efficacy. They know they will have to make many fewer decisions and as a result, fewer mistakes are possible, and if it doesn't work out, then—well, someone or something is available to blame. Why struggle with the risks of learning to motivate from within? To stay with external motivation (commercial help) and to go with an easier way to get the job done is a strong message to the self not to trust or believe in that self.

In my earlier book, *Change Your Mind: Change Your Weight*, I speak of the path to self-motivation which starts with desire, something which may be lacking in a depressed person. However, even if this most basic impulse is missing, it is usually temporary. Because we have eyes, ears, and a brain that is able to imagine things in response to the stimuli of the environment, we are vulnerable to new possibilities that establish desire anew. When we want something, we are open to seeing possibilities. Once we can see possibilities, we begin to see how we might attain our goal. We can take something that is possible and see it as probable, and this creates hope. When we hope, we can sense our goal within our reach. Now, how do we make that last step to get hold of what we are after?

At this point, we are still in an action phase, and this is where the individual effort may break down. This occurs just before we get to the top of the hill. Except for the initial desire which came from inside, up to this point, external motivation has provided the power. Please remember that what we are after is a change in our own behavior. People often get this confused with thinking they need to focus on a loss of pounds, rather than on the attitudes (beliefs) that lead to the behavior changes that will result in the loss of the pounds.

If the focus of what we are attempting to obtain (a lasting change in certain behaviors and ultimately a more self-efficacious view of ourselves) is not kept clear, we will get into trouble at this point. Also, if our motivation does not become an internal drive but rather remains external (e.g., commercial weight loss programs, services, gurus, products, etc.) we will quickly be right back at the starting point of desire.

With an internal focus to gain greater self-awareness and clarity of one's own beliefs and value priorities, decisions are simpler and personal freedom is accepted. If we accept that we are free to be who we want to be, it is much harder to find excuses and to place blame for not changing. The difficulty at this point is finding the courage to take the risks inherent in actively, deliberately, and consciously changing.

Once the action of change has been experienced on a continuum, we tend to believe what we have seen ourselves do. Watching ourselves take the action and risk and achieving periodic gains, we come to believe we can count on ourselves to come through. Self-confidence and self-trust grow, and we are less likely to procrastinate about the next effort. Better yet, we realize we don't need to look to an outside provider for motivation.

Again, the answer lies in the problem. What we avoid doing because it is hard, is the very thing that changes our perception of ourselves and thus changes our inaction to action.

SUMMARY

Dr. David McClelland, the prominent Harvard professor who has researched motivation for more than forty years, provides many insights in his book, *Human Motivation* (Cambridge Univ. Press, 1985). He indicates a clear element of subconscious motivation in all humans, including people like Louise, but he also discusses research which shows that we are aware of most of our motives. Dr. McClelland speaks of four major motive systems: achievement, power, affiliation, and avoidance, all of which seem to be tied into the understanding of the chronically overweight person. There are many different influences on motivation, from biological influences of smell and taste memories or sex, to unlimited factors of social or environmental conditioning. Even those of us with a high degree of self-awareness do not immediately see the connection between all the different motivational factors and their influences to our immediate urges. Understanding why we procrastinate about exercising or why we feel a need to eat when our stomach is already full requires a truly involved effort to determine our stronger, basic underlying drives. It also requires an exploration of our ever-shifting motivations and our ever-shifting experiences and environmental influences.

Confused? Who wouldn't be? The more one becomes involved with the academic research, the different theories, the means of measuring motivation, and the bringing of the multiple variables of multiple personal motivations together, the more confusing it can become. Reading or counseling with professionals who are able to be objective may be helpful in speeding up the process; however, in the final analysis, each of us will have to determine the ultimate truth of why we don't do what seems logical or why we do what is often self-defeating in our own lives.

We do have similarities with certain groups of people that practice behaviors similar to our own, and we can learn from them, as was discussed earlier in Chapter 9 about the 5-Plus Club. However, we are still unique individuals with unique circumstances that are constantly changing. The best part is that we have a large degree of free choice to influence our own life, which includes even our motivations.

Learning how we can best motivate our change through our own insights into ourselves and the practice of those elements which give our lives a degree of peace, health, and self-efficacy certainly will lead to a life that is full, stimulating, are satisfying, and that indeed is an adventure that includes more harmony than discord. Excessive fat rarely accompanies a life that is intrinsically motivated.

To see ourselves clearly, we must be calm and feel safe enough to be able to focus on what we have learned by observation, listening, and experience. To feel calm and safe over extended periods of time we must believe we can trust ourselves to get up and try again after we have fallen (risk taking) in our efforts to learn and grow. By following through on our practice of mastery, understanding and living out a wellness lifestyle, and practicing the consistency of empowerment behaviors leads to the intrinsic motivation required for long-term, successful, balanced weight that requires effort but little or no mental struggles or conflict called procrastination.

Chapter 14

EMPOWERMENT

Moving from "Control" to Harmony

*T*he faces looking up at me are full of hope, insight and understanding seconds after completing my six-hour workshop with only one break per three-hour stretch. I am feeling very stimulated and self-satisfied (i.e., smug), not only because I was able to hold the audience's attention, but also because the message appears to have gotten through. I've talked about the futility of weight loss diets, the importance of risk taking for long-term change, moving from external to internal motivation, getting beyond procrastination, and letting go of the quest for magical, easy answers as the first step to long-term success.

Then someone bursts my balloon of pride and hope with a single question that lets me know the point of the six-hour seminar has been missed.

This scene has been played out many times, not only with my workshops but also after hour-long pre-program interviews in my office designed to give prospective new clients a realistic perspective. The questions that I find so devastating usually go something like: "How many calories are there in your diet?" or, "What things should I do before the next session?" or the classic, "Do I have to exercise before I lose enough weight to look good in my exercise outfit?"

What they have let me know is that they are still counting on me, or on the program, product or book, to change them—i.e., that changing self-doubt isn't their goal, and learning to take risks and face discomfort are not what they came to me for. Reading the book, coming to group, and following the plan are okay for awhile, but working on recognizing the underlying causes and taking the risks required for self-change are difficult and frightening, and that is when the whole weight loss-through-wellness scheme breaks down, even in the most comprehensive and healthiest of programs.

After twenty years of trying to nurture self-efficacy using every means known to me, I have realized that the more comprehensive and structured the program, the more it costs, the more charismatic the leader, the more gimmicks and products it uses, and the longer the participants stay with "the program," the *less* likely it is that meaningful, long-term, intrinsic change will come about and/or, in this case, the less likely it is that weight loss will occur. Telling people not to look outside of themselves, but rather to look within themselves for answers is a contradiction when they have paid $3,000, have a respected professional guiding them and a bunch of other people around them looking for the same magic answer—and they are experiencing it all in a facility devoted to "curing illness."

You may be wondering why, then, I even wrote this book: isn't it just another means to encourage people to continue seeking the magic? But this book has no magic—instead it explores how to find the magic *inside yourself.* This book is written only for individuals who want to find a direction where, if they will look, work, and take risks, they can bring about not only a healthful weight balance but also a confidant harmony inside themselves. A book or a tape won't change you or the belief you have in yourself, but it will give you information about how you can bring change about when you are ready. Louise is a good example of how one person can bring about her own changes.

WHAT EVER HAPPENED TO LOUISE?

After the Weight Loss through Wellness program ended and my research started, Louise became a part of my experimental, leaderless support group for change which ran for three months. During that period, Louise started a follow-through effort that went very well for a month, then tapered off and stopped. The leaderless group seemed to help at first, but it quickly faded away. It almost seemed like the more the group bonded, the less action was taken by most of the group members. It wasn't until several weeks after the group ended that Louise began to progress like never before.

It was a beautiful fall Saturday, and Louise was waiting for a friend across from a public park. As she sat in her car she noticed a group of people in the park exercising together—practicing a movement exercise she had learned about in the wellness program. As she watched the group, it seemed more like a choreographed dance than an exercise. The group completely captured her attention, and she quickly became enraptured with the beauty of the movements. Her busy, worried mind seem to quiet down and do nothing more than focus on the movements. Louise realized a deep calm had come over her when her friend arrived, touched her and asked if anything was wrong. It was a new and wonderful experience, and it was no surprise to find Louise a part of the exercise group the following Saturday.

Tai chi chuan is the exercise Louise became attracted to. It is a Chinese martial art form that requires complete attention in order to become skilled in it. Louise valued it first as a way of quieting her mind and delivering the sense of peace she felt whenever she practiced, but it also gave her a feeling of connection with everything around her and a clarity in her thinking. If it had given her nothing else, she would have continued her training. She did not feel particularly skilled in tai chi, but as time went on, she did develop her movements to the point where her teacher asked her to take part in a group demonstration.

This both excited and frightened Louise at the same time. She practiced extremely hard in the days before the event. Then the day before her performance, she pulled a muscle in her back and was unable to take part in the demonstration. Her teacher told her she was trying too hard to be the best, and that she only needed to keep practicing her routines over and over to reach excellence and learn patience. Louise wondered if she had subconsciously sabotaged herself as a way to avoid the pressure of possible failure.

Weeks passed, and her teacher did not ask her to take part in the next several demonstrations. Some practice days, Louise felt like she was making little or no progress, and sometimes she didn't want to practice at all. She would go to practice anyway, go through the same familiar motions and leave practice mellow and energetic, and happy that she had taken part. Gradually she forgot about the demonstrations and, except for a few missed practices, soon she had spent a year just going through the movements. Then after practice one Saturday, the teacher asked her if she would take part in a demonstration at a very large and special conference. She hadn't thought about it for so long it took her by surprise but, flattered, she said she would. She remembered what her instructor had said, "just stay with your usual routine."

This time it all came off beautifully. Louise knew she had reached a new level in her tai chi, but she also knew she had come to enjoy the simple practice more than reaching a recognized level of mastery. She knew if she were to reach still higher levels, they would come when she had put in much more time simply going through the basic movements, and that pushing and straining to make it happen faster would only be counter-productive.

In that year of practice, Louise had also started to exhibit many of the characteristics identified with the members of the 5-Plus Club. She was changing her life and her habits, and she had stopped struggling with herself, with her husband, and with her work. Louise, the consummate perfectionist, no longer needed to control and manipulate her way through life. Eating for health was now an adventure, and her newly developing capacities in aerobic exercise excited her. Louise was starting to focus on her own intrinsic motivations for day-to-day decisions, but most importantly, she trusted herself more with each new day. She had been living up to her own values because she saw herself go through long periods of time staying true to her practice when it was hard, inconvenient, and especially when she felt she was making little or no progress. She knew, now, that she could count on *Louise* which made it much easier to face her fears, especially the fear of possibly failing.

Louise had allowed herself to become involved with a discipline in a way very different from compliance to weight loss diets and exercise routines. This time she had not sought the instant gratification of dropping forty pounds. She was not after any greater goal than the joy of the movement and the satisfaction of practicing the process. This time it wasn't a matter of control and forcing herself through each practice to achieve praise; she practiced because she wanted to—even when her improvements over long periods of time were very slow. Breakthroughs occurred when they were not expected, and Louise became more skillful, but that wasn't the point.

The longer Louise practiced, the more she found a calmness that was never there when she struggled to meet the expectations of a weight loss effort. She also became more sensitive to her own feelings and found changes occurring in most other areas of her life. She was starting to believe in herself and the fact that the goals came as a by-product of her efforts along the way.

Problems relating to eating, exercise, relationships, sex, etc., were still there, but not to the degree they once were. Fears still came up and she didn't like them any better, but the way she dealt with them was more effective and direct. She did not react to them by overeating. Louise had turned her focus inward and balanced it with her outward focus. Her answers about how to deal with her environment were within herself, and not to be found from the magic weight loss programs. She no longer doubted herself. She knew she would make mistakes, and she also knew she would recover from them. "Control" was no longer necessary.

Louise is not fully where she wants to be yet and is happy to know she never will be. She has learned that challenges are valuable and not to be afraid of them. The practice of tai chi will bring her new levels of achievement and praise, but it is the practice itself that she loves; and she can like herself for bringing the changes about. Louise's impatient struggle has stopped, she is learning that the practice is more valuable than the excellence and praise it brings. Oh, yes—most of the weight is off and she has no doubts about the rest coming or that she will be able to keep it off. Conquering her weight is no longer a struggle. Louise is learning she will be whatever she wants to be.

Earl, Louise's husband, has more than noticed the changes—not just in her weight, but in the way she uses her time, the comfortable attitude she has about people, and her confidence in herself. Earl knows he has some decisions to make about himself now. Louise has moved to a different, healthier place. Does he want to move on, too, or continue to be separated from her and her life? Even if he does change and grow, he may grow in a different direction. He realizes that it is what he wants for himself that is important. If he gets to a better place with his own life, it can only improve his relationship with Louise, even if it only means they part better friends. What he hasn't considered yet is that no person stands still in life, he either grows and changes or he moves backwards. Both forward and back are risky, but only forward offers hope.

Louise has a momentum going now—an energy and a belief in herself that is building and can carry her through each new problem and fear. Her back may never be perfect, and her work may be filled with peaks and valleys, but she has learned she has the magic inside herself to carry her along with a quality to her life that makes it worth living.

DOING IT ON YOUR OWN

Doing it on your own is just that—doing it alone. Can you solicit support? Yes, in the same way you talk about your day when you come home in the evening. It is never really possible to avoid making your own decisions and owning responsibility for them if you want to take credit for the outcomes. This does not mean you can never learn from others or listen to their opinions. All kinds of resources can be brought into this process, but without the risk of self-initiated action to experience what you believe you understand, you will have no emotional integration in your beliefs about yourself. In other words, you would continue to perceive yourself as you have, with self-doubt and low self-esteem.

Control or Harmony?

Most commonly encountered methods, techniques, or practices to bring about change in emotions, behavior, or self-concept tend to be "magic" from others that will require no risk taking and no confronting of all the frightening possibilities. Also, at the same time, by even seeking magic, we reinforce feelings of self-doubt and reduce self-esteem. How to handle this difficult, frightening dilemma and what Louise has been doing through her mastery of tai chi is what this chapter is about.

Ironically, in some ways we are seeking that which we already are—nothing more than being ourselves. I mean truly being who we are without any covers, pretenses, or fears of not meeting the expectations we think others have for us. It often seems too risky in a competitive "winner-loser" world to live by our own beliefs, values, and intuitive decisions after a lifetime of being rewarded for pleasing others and trying to make ourselves lovable instead of learning how to love.

Taking the chance of leaping that chasm where we disconnect from the familiar and go hurdling through that unknown space, trying to find an orientation to begin anew without dropping into the abyss or smashing into a rocky wall, but touching down gently to make a successful new beginning on the other side, is often perceived as too risky. This change, this risky leap, can be facilitated by some insights and understanding—maybe even some practice. The risk, the decisions, the action, the ending of what you were hanging on to that kept you overweight and frightened, confronting the fear of reorientating, and starting anew must be your own. If you do not experience yourself going through this process, you will have no emotional integration of what you have come to understand intellectually. In an attempt to avoid risk, fearful people seek control through such things as structured, organized diets and programs. These efforts almost always prove to backfire.

Control, as has been mentioned in other chapters, does not seem to be effective in the long term for bringing about change. With the small percentage of those who bring about long-term change by attempting to control themselves and their environment, the experience is one of a great deal of on-going stress and inner conflict. Some proponents of control methods have a saying that sums up the problem very well, "live one day at a time." Whether controlling is external or strictly an internal struggle, the results seem to be about the same. The difference between control and harmony is analogous to dancing to music by envisioning the foot marks on the floor and counting the steps with the beat versus moving to the rhythm of the music as you feel it and your body naturally responds to it, without the fear of taking a wrong step.

In Louise's case, she went from trying to have others control her (which didn't work) to trying to structure and control herself (which didn't work) to finding harmony through a discipline (which did work). How and why did this happen? Wasn't she still receiving assistance?

An old country western song has a line which seems appropriate, "I long for the freedom of my chains." In other words, once Louise chose a direction for herself and gave it a purpose and meaning; she was no longer just a leaf blowing in the wind. Each new weight loss program or product had lasted until a stronger wind caught her attention. When she chose a direction for herself, she exercised her freedom. Now, she was not just being blown by the wind, she had become a part of it; blending and flowing together with it in harmony. Because she made a choice for herself, she has no need to rebel. Her energy can be used to move with the new direction instead of resisting it. Louise can now use the wind to lift her and carry her where she wants to go.

Because Louise is engaged in a harmonious effort, the struggle in her mind is no longer there—she prefers what she has chosen to do. Each time she practices again, she believes in her ability to choose, her inner trust grows, and her self-doubt wanes. With her continued practice, she also believes more strongly in her abilities to focus and guide her body as she wishes and move her emotions to the center. With continued practice, she has more peak experiences, and she comes to value the practice and patience as much as she values reaching the peak. With the struggle turned into a preference and the finding of harmony in other new, self-chosen directions, her life transitions have become smoother. With each new transition, life is less threatening. Inner security grows, and centeredness is increased, bringing out the best in her, which in turn builds her confidence, skills, insights, relationships, intellect, creativity, and general happiness as the conditions of her life (which she used to blame for her problems) continue to rise and fall without Louise falling apart (e.g., regaining her weight).

Is Tai Chi the Answer for You?

Louise happens to be using tai chi chuan as a discipline to master; however, it could just as easily be some other already established discipline, or one that she created herself. Dr. George Leonard (author of *Mastery: The Keys to Success and Long-Term Fulfillment*) discusses the martial art form called aikido but, as he indicates, it isn't for everybody. Also, if disciplines such as martial arts, meditation, or yoga are too esoteric or too difficult to identify with, try something closer to your current interests and values. Activities that you believe add to your health or contribute in some way to a better world bring with them additional psychological and motivational benefits, and they may serve you best.

Painting, knitting, dancing, carpentry, biking, gardening, public speaking, or playing an instrument are just a few examples of activities that can be used to work toward mastery of a discipline. What is important is that you choose; that you allow yourself to be fully engrossed and consistent with what you choose; and that you approach it in such a manner that you don't try to control it, but rather allow yourself to find harmony with it.

EMPOWERMENT: OUTCOME OR ALTERNATIVE TO MASTERY?

Empowerment is a buzz word and can be one result of working at mastery, or something that is worked at in a more direct, cognitive manner. To empower yourself is to give yourself the means to achieve self-efficacy. *Self-efficacy* is the conviction that you can successfully change your behavior to reach your goals. Empowerment, like mastery, is a method of changing your self-image and raising your self-esteem, something that chronically overweight people tend to lose sight of in their impatient rush to lose weight. Co-dependency groups and business management consultants are strongly pushing the concept of empowerment at this time, and even some political and school reform movements emphasize empowerment to raise self-esteem for children and parents, and to help employees to feel a sense of ownership with their jobs and life responsibilities. Compulsive behaviors can indicate the lack of empowerment attitudes.

Here are some of the practices involved in self-empowerment:

- A *commitment* to stick with your vision through the easy and hard times is a must. This means a commitment which has such a high priority on your list of values that very few, if any, other values will supersede it. A clarity of exactly what the commitment includes is required so that it won't be ignored in the midst of the distractions of day-to-day decisions.

- A *discipline* to learn to follow through on the commitment is equally important, as shown in Dr. Leonard's *Mastery* and the way it served Louise. Remember, discipline that works is achieved through harmony.

- *Relationships* dedicated to supporting personal growth certainly contributed in a major way to the long-term success of the 5-Plus Club Members. A friendship, spouse, siblings, even kids for whom you are a role model, or professionals who also serve as friends can all be a part of the support with which you sustain your effort. Again, be very clear on exactly what is supportive to personal growth and how to adjust it when changes or good intentions have gone awry. Also, it will be extremely important to reach down deep for the courage inside when you don't think it is there, and when you think your fear of staying on track is about to overwhelm you. Please don't forget to give yourself credit (a mental pat on the back) when you are afraid to do something and you do it anyway.

- *Spontaneity and intuition* will serve you much better in the long run than having a structured plan devised for you. You need a sense of your body and what it needs—not just a calorie count to force yourself to stick to. A quick decision to get out of bed for that early morning jog rather than a long mental struggle about the pros and cons of getting started or staying in bed works better. Some decisions about where you want to go are not always clear or easy, and your gut-level intuition usually provides a good sense of what will work—so learn to trust it. Practicing being in touch with your feelings at the time you feel them will help immensely. Knowing what you are telling yourself and imaging in your mind at any given moment will also be of great help to your intention. Practice monitoring these aspects of yourself until it is natural for you to always be in touch with how you are influencing yourself without a conscious deliberate effort.

- *Humor and play* can get you through the hard times and beyond your emotional burdens. They provide the balance you are looking for in your life as a whole. Humor and play are natural, and whenever you are not too intense, you give them space to come out. It is part of the child in you and it is where your creativity and imagination reside. Humor and play are very practical when you think about it. Norman Cousins, the great writer, believes humor is what saved him from a terminal illness and a heart attack, and he has written several books on the subject. Most of all, humor and play help us to know we are alive and turn what could be depressing life and work situations into fun. They support the positive attitudes that lead to discovering our full potentials to not only succeed but to thrive.

- *Nurturing self-worth* essentially means you become as important to yourself as the importance you place on the needs, expectations, and requests of others. Nurturing self-worth means being responsible to others by being responsible for yourself. Taking enough of your own time, energy, thought, and other means to bring your health and well-being to a point where you realize the benefits of these priorities, not only for your own physical and emotional well-being, but because you see that love, acceptance and respect from others also comes with it. In taking care of yourself, you also have a greater and wiser capacity when you do give to others. Nurturing self-worth is risk-taking because you do take your time and attention away from those from whom you fear rejection. It often brings feelings of guilt as well, until you start recognizing your own worth. Without going through this practice, all the other empowerment practices will be for naught.

- *Ownership of responsibility* for who and what you are as a person, the feelings you generate, the behavior you choose, the beliefs you hold, and your responses to your life experiences is what self-empowerment is all about. How you accept the ownership—be it with desire or trepidation, reluctance or enthusiasm—makes a great difference as to the satisfaction of ownership. It belongs to you; it always has, and it always will—whether you want it or not. It is your freedom to be what you want to be or a huge burden to carry for life. Every personal growth theory is aimed at each person accepting this ownership, because it is where you have the best chance to thrive.

- *Changing* (adjusting) to the experiences of your life as they happen is necessary to finding harmony. Trying to stay the same as the world around you changes or as time and experience changes what goes on within you is like trying to hold the river with your hands: not only is it impossible, you are overwhelmed or become so exhausted you simply let go and get pushed backward. You don't stand still but are always moving forward or backward. For some people, the choice of learning to let go or relax is the first step forward.

- *Full spectrum perspective* of your life and the world you live in is essential, especially in dealing with perfectionist details. A global vision gives you balance. If you have full spectrum perspective when looking at your flat tire on a hot day when you are dressed for an important appointment for which you are about to be late, you are able to see your life in total—that is, all you have lived and all you have left to live. In that moment, the situation is seen as the very small part of your life that it is. With this perspective, you are able to handle problems better, recover from them more quickly, and laugh about them later with a minimum of distress.

Empowerment, then, is something you always had available that you now give to yourself. It is an attitude you choose and a way of viewing yourself and your world that allows for the best of whatever you are to be realized. Like mastery, it brings you to a less conflicted and more harmonious, balanced centeredness where extremes, such as obesity, do not exist. You can give to yourself a relaxed energy that can be used and not wasted on wheel-spinning.

WEIGHT LOSS THROUGH WELLNESS

Like empowerment, the wellness lifestyle is still more involved, and can be approached more directly than the mastery used by Louise. This method can include many aspects of well-being which can be broken into many different categories. This is a more academic and intellectual approach that is simply based on the accumulation of appropriate information and the application of that information. The loss of weight or

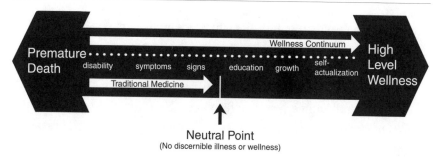

The Wellness Continuum.

maintaining healthful weight balance need not have anything directly to do with the intended purpose of achieving a wellness lifestyle; those concerns will be adjusted as a natural by-product of living the wellness lifestyle. With mastery, the focus is on the practice of the discipline. In empowerment, the focus is on the understanding, development, and practice of a self-enhancing attitude. The focus of this method is health (wellness). How healthy can you be? On one side of a total health scale, humans may fall into levels of illness ("worseness") with anything from a hangnail to premature death. At the center we have the absence of illness—a body without disease, mind and body parts that are not malfunctioning in any observable way, a neutral point beyond which are levels of wellness. For a great many people this is an area that is totally unexplored and, as you can see on the scale above, it holds the potential of many untapped riches.

The weight loss through wellness method can be categorized in many ways, and no matter how the many aspects of it are organized, there is no set order that is right for everyone. This is especially true considering how our needs keep changing, and only the person who experiences the needs has the potential to be aware of what is needed at any given moment. Ownership of wellness cannot be given away. Therefore, the following eight steps to self-change and growth are meant to be completed in the order and speed that best suits the needs of each individual user. Several steps could be worked on at once, or they could be worked on one at a time.

Before starting on any one aspect of each of the eight steps, it may be useful to pick out those areas which are the most urgent and those that are in the least urgent need of attention as a way of getting started. The eight steps start and end with belief (philosophy of life). Your persistence and determination in completing all eight steps will earn you the belief in yourself. As in all cases of self-change, *you are the boss*.

Although my earlier book, *Change Your Mind: Change Your Weight*, covers all the aspects indicated here in greater detail, you may need to seek still greater detail from other local resources. Your initiation in finding the information and taking action as you feel a need for it is a crucial factor in bringing about the changes you seek.

A GRADUAL PROCESS

Step I

Self-awareness: In the long term, self-awareness deals with identifying the underlying causes that can make individuals vulnerable to becoming more easily stressed, more strongly stressed, and having stress last longer. Some on-going causes of stress often include the need for:

- Belief clarification
- Value-priority rankings
- Decisions to achieve self-esteem, and
- Understanding the whole person and existential self.

In the short term, self-awareness has to do with the minute-to-minute situations of each day and how we generate our own emotions or handle the emotions we have created based on what we experience and our perceived ability to cope with those perceptions. These factors are:

- Monitoring self-talk
- Monitoring mental pictures
- Monitoring emotions, and
- Cognitive modification of perfectionist behaviors and thinking.

Step II

Health, fitness and nutrition:

- Learn healthful eating and exercise practices

- Develop a sensitivity to your body's needs
- Develop healthful taste and exercise practice preferences through a gradual (no resistance) process, and
- Educate yourself regarding medical self-care education, and accept responsibility for your treatment decisions

Step III

Emotional ownership:

- Learn and practice daily stress reduction techniques
- Utilize behavioral self-ownership options, and
- Build a support system

Step IV

Communication skills:

- Be open, honest and tactful in expression of feelings
- Clarify your thoughts
- Recognize when you make rationalizations and when you are manipulating others
- Develop assertiveness
- Develop voice power and body language skills

Step V

Self-image building:

- Acknowledge and identify fears
- Desensitization of fears and risk taking
- Social adventures
- What has meaning/purpose, or leads to aliveness

Step VI

Environment/community involvement:

- Learn and practice a sound ecology for everyone
- Learn and practice keeping personal food, water, home, and workplace clean and unpolluted
- Contribute to improvement in socio/political/economic well-being for everyone

Step VII

Peak experiences: Seek availability to total harmony with all aspects of your life, including the:

- Physical
- Intellectual
- Social
- Psychological
- Spiritual
- Play/Humor

Step VIII

Ownership of personal freedom (existential reality): Learn and practice through:

- Choice/decision making
- Commitment
- Awareness
- Responsibility
- Experiencing
- Initiating
- Intrinsic motivation

- Self-actualization (becoming the better self as you believe that to be)

- Transcending self

- Meaning (satisfaction with your motion) which comes from: 1) What you give to life; 2) What you take from life; 3) the stand you take toward your condition (including the tragic triad of existence, pain, death, guilt).

You can focus on and practice *mastery*, *empowerment,* and the *wellness lifestyle* separately, and yet it will lead to the same end. Each method blends into the others at some point, and harmony will be attained by anyone who chooses to persist with any of the three. Individuals who achieve long-term success on their own most often use some parts or all of these methods of change.

How or if one defines these methods is relatively unimportant compared to the personal desire to bring about change. Each person seems to have his or her own strength, purpose, and beliefs which will be directed where necessary as the need for adjustment in each new situation arises. The method that you choose and own as yours is the one you will permit to work for you.

In the end, the answers reside within you.

Appendix A

COOKBOOKS AND OTHER RESOURCES

Akers, Keith: *A Vegetarian Sourcebook: The Nutrition, Ecology and Ethics of a Natural Foods Diet.* Baltimore, MD: Vegetarian Resource Group, 1993.

Csikszentimihaly, Mihaly: *Finding Flow.* New York: Basic Books, 1988.

Davis, Gail, and Neil Bernard: *The Complete Guide to Vegetarian Convenience Foods.* Troutdale, OR: NewSage Press, 1999.

Hagler, Louise: *Tofu Cookery.* Summertown, TN: Book Pub. Co., 1991.

Geiskopf-Hadler, Susann, and Mindy Toomay: *The Vegan Gourmet: Expanded Second Edition.* Roseville, CA: Prima Publishing, 1999.

Grogan, Bryanna Clark: *Soyfoods Cooking for a Positive Menopause.* Summertown, TN: Book Pub. Co., 1999.

Grogan, Bryanna Clark: *20 Minutes to Dinner: Quick, Low-Fat, Low-Calorie Vegetarian Meals.* Summertown, TN: Book Pub. Co., 1997.

Leneman, Leah: *The Single Vegan: Simple, Convenient and Appetizing Meals for One.* New York: Thorson's Pub., 1989.

Leonard, George: *Mastery: The Keys to Success and Long-Term Fulfillment.* New York: Plume, 1992.

McClelland, David: *Human Motivation.* Boston: Cambridge University Press, 1988.

Peele, Stanton: *Diseasing of America: Addiction Treatment Out of Control*. Lanham, MD: Lexington Books, 1989.

Raymond, Joanne: *The Peaceful Palate: Fine Vegetarian Cuisine*. Summertown, TN: Book Pub. Co., 1996.

Robbins, John, and Johanna Macy: *Diet for a New America: How Your Food Choices Affect Your Health, Happiness and the Future of Life on Earth*. Tiburon, CA: HJ Kramer, 1999.

Robbins, John, and Jeanne Marie Martin. *Vegan Delights*. Madeira Park, BC: Harbour Publishing Co., 1987.

Schinner, Miyoko Nishimoto: *Japanese Cooking: Contemporary and Traditional—Simple, Delicious, and Vegan*. Summertown, TN: Book Pub. Co., 1999.

Solomon, Jay: *150 Vegan Favorites: Fresh, Easy and Incredibly Delicious Recipes You Can Enjoy Every Day*. Roseville, CA: Prima Publishing, 1998.

Stepaniak, Joanne: *Delicious Food for a Healthy Heart*. Summertown, TN: Book Pub. Co., 1999.

Stepaniak, Joanne: *Vegan Vittles: Recipes Inspired by the Critters at Farm Sanctuary*. Summertown, TN: Book Pub Co., 1996.

Stepaniak, Joanne, and Virginia Messina: *The Vegan Sourcebook*. Los Angeles, CA: Lowell House, 1998.

Wasserman, Debra: *Conveniently Vegan: Turn Packaged Foods into Delicious Vegetarian Dishes*. Baltimore, MD: Vegetarian Resource Group, 1997.

Wasserman, Debra: *Simply Vegan: Quick Vegetarian Meals*. Baltimore, MD: Vegetarian Resource Group, 1999.

Wasserman, Debra, and Reed Mangels (eds.): *The Vegan Handbook: Over 200 Delicious Recipes, Meal Plans and Vegetarian Resources for All Ages*. Baltimore, MD: Vegetarian Resource Group, 1996.

Wasserman, Debra, and Charles Stahler: *Meatless Meals for Working People: Quick and Easy Vegetarian Recipes, Second Edition.* Baltimore, MD: Vegetarian Resource Group, 1998.

Weil, Andrew: *Eating Well for Optimum Health.* New York: Alfred A. Knopf, 2000.

Appendix B

UNDERSTAND YOUR BLOOD TEST

Please note that this appendix is intended to be used only as an aid. It is not *a substitute for a professional medical interpretation. For a detailed, personalized explanation of your blood test, see your family physician.*

ALBUMIN

Average Range: 3.0 - 5.5 g/dl

Albumin is a form of high quality protein that is synthesized in the liver. Decreased blood levels may indicate chronic liver disease or a diet that is deficient in protein.

ALK PHOSPHATASE

Average Range: 51 - 227 U/L

Alkaline phosphatase is an enzyme, which is a substance that helps speed up chemical reactions in the body. Because this particular enzyme is normally found in bone and liver tissue, high blood levels can indicate problems with these areas of the body. Low levels of alkaline phosphatase are fairly rare, but can sometimes point to a dietary deficiency in vitamin C.

ALT (SGPT) (ALANINE AMINOTRANSFERASE / SERUM GLUTAMIC-PYRUVIC TRANSAMINASE)

Average Range: 3 - 35 U/L

This enzyme is found mainly in the liver. Thus, a high level of SPGT is an accurate indicator of liver disease or injury. By comparing these results with those of other enzyme tests, it is possible for your doctor to more readily determine sources of enzyme release in the body.

AST (SGOT) (ASPARTATE AMINOTRANSFERASE / SERUM GLUTAMIC-OXALOACETIC TRANSAMINASE)

Average Range: 7 - 37 U/L

This is an enzyme which is present primarily in the heart muscle and liver, but is also found in common muscle tissue, the kidneys, and red blood cells. Test results above the normal range can indicate tissue injury involving any of these areas of the body.

BUN (BLOOD UREA NITROGEN)

Average Range: 5 - 25 mg/dl

This is a kidney function test that measures how well nitrogen waste, the end product of protein metabolism, is being filtered from the blood stream. Scores above the normal range may indicate kidney or prostate problems.

CALCIUM

Average Range: 8.4 - 10.4 mg/dl

Calcium is a mineral important for bone formation, muscle contraction, and blood clotting. Abnormal calcium levels can signify a variety of potential problems. For instance, low levels of blood calcium may result from underactive thyroid and/or parathyroid glands, a tendency to hyperventilate, problems with the pancreas, or a vitamin D deficiency. Conversely, high levels of calcium in the blood may indicate bone disease, excessive calcium intake (e.g., milk), an overconsumption of vitamin D or of high protein foods (e.g., meats), the most common reason for calcium loss from the bones.

CARBON DIOXIDE

Average Range: 23 - 32 mEg/L

This test is used to assess the acid-base levels (pH) of the blood. High levels of carbon dioxide can result from such things as lung disease, intestinal problems (vomiting, diarrhea) or the use of diuretics (water pills). Conversely, low levels of carbon dioxide can indicate such things as uncontrolled diabetes, kidney problems, or a tendency to hyperventilate.

CHLORIDE

Average Range: 95 - 110 mEg/L

Like sodium and potassium, chloride is an important electrolyte that serves many essential bodily functions. An unusually high chloride reading can suggest kidney malfunction, whereas a low level of blood chloride tends to develop in conjunction with low levels of potassium.

CHOLESTEROL

Average Range: 70 - 199 mg/dl
HDL: 35 - 999 mg/dl
LDL: 0 - 129 mg/dl

Cholesterol is an important blood chemical that is necessary for fat digestion, hormone production, and healthy skin. Lower than normal levels of cholesterol may indicate poor dietary habits, liver disease, or an overactive thyroid. Conversely, unusually high levels of blood cholesterol can signal problems with the liver, pancreas or kidneys. High cholesterol levels have also been linked to heart attacks and strokes. These risks can be reduced by decreasing consumption of red meats, rich dairy products and fried foods.

CREATININE

Average Range: 0.7 - 1.4 mg/dl

Like the BUN test, the creatinine test also measures the ability of the kidneys to filter a waste product from the blood. Because creatinine is the by-product of a high energy compound found in muscle tissue, persons with greater muscle mass may tend to have slightly elevated levels of blood creatinine.

GGT (GAMMA-GLUTAMYLTRANSPEPTIDASE)

Average Range: 9 - 65 U/L

This is another enzyme that is found primarily in the liver. The test is sensitive to detecting excessive levels of alcohol consumption, which can cause the liver to release this enzyme into the bloodstream. Elevated GGT levels can also suggest liver disease or gall bladder problems.

GLUCOSE

Average Range: 65 - 110 mg/dl

This is primarily a test for diabetes, which may be indicated by a high level of glucose in the blood. It shows how well the body handles carbohydrate metabolism. Glucose may be burned directly or stored as fat. High blood glucose levels can also result from extreme stress, an overactive thyroid, or excessive release of adrenaline. Low glucose levels may suggest an underactive pituitary gland, or problems with the pancreas (hypoglycemia).

LDH (LACTATE DEHYDROGENASE)

Average Range: 100 - 225 U/L

This blood test measures an enzyme normally found in the heart, liver, brain, muscles and red blood cells. Although this particular test cannot pinpoint the exact problem area of enzyme release, another form of the LDH test is available which can distinguish among the five primary sources of LDH released into the bloodstream.

PHOSPHOROUS

Average Range: 2.5 - 4.5 mg/dl

Blood levels of phosphorous are highly dependent upon blood calcium levels; and vice versa. Thus, many of the problems suggested by abnormal calcium are also implicated by abnormal phosphorous levels. Beyond serving to confirm results of the calcium test, a high phosphorous level can indicate kidney problems. Also, high phosphorous readings are sometimes due to an excessive intake of red meat, soft drinks, and junk food.

POTASSIUM

Average Range: 3.5 - 5.3 mEg/L

High levels of blood serum potassium can signify problems with the kidneys, pituitary gland, or adrenal glands. Conversely, low blood potassium levels can result from diuretic therapy, insufficient magnesium, liver disease, use of certain hormones and/or steroids, chronic stress, a poor diet, chronic diarrhea, and chronic fever with perspiration. Deficiencies in potassium can also lead to muscle fatigue and weakness in the legs and arms.

SODIUM

Average Range: 135 - 146 mEg/L

Low sodium levels are fairly uncommon and sometimes indicative of a head injury, dehydration, or high steroid levels. High blood sodium is more commonly encountered. This may indicate a heavy use of laxatives, vomiting, diarrhea, heat stress, or a poor diet.

TOTAL BILIRUBIN

Average Range: 0.0 - 1.1 mg/dl

Bilirubin is a waste product that results from the natural destruction of red blood cells. Under normal circumstances, bilirubin is carried to the liver where it is process for blood filtering by the kidneys. Thus, high levels of bilirubin in the blood may indicate problems associated with the liver (e.g., hepatitis) or conditions influencing the number of red blood cells (e.g., infection or anemia).

TOTAL PROTEIN

Average Range: 6.0 - 8.0 g/dl

The liver is the site of protein synthesis and production. Therefore, the level of protein detected in the blood provides a good indication of overall liver functioning. A low level of total blood protein may also indicate a poor nutritional intake of protein-rich foods.

TRIGLYCERIDES

Average Range: 35 - 160 mg/dl

This test measures a type of fat in the blood that results from overuse of sugar or alcohol, or from obesity. As compared to cholesterol, this is a relatively minor factor in coronary risk. Furthermore, triglyceride levels can usually be reduced through weight reduction.

URIC ACID

Average Range: 3.5 - 8.0 mg/dl

High blood levels of uric acid are often an indication of a tendency to develop gout and/or the presence of kidney stones. Acid is an end product of the body's metabolism. Also, high levels of uric acid in the blood can provide another indication of poor kidney functioning.

INDEX

ABOUT THE AUTHOR

*J*ames McClernan, Ed.D., is a licensed psychologist, with twelve years of hospital-based experience researching, designing, and conducting weight programs. He is the author of two books and over forty articles dealing with this subject and has appeared on hundreds of media interviews.

Dr. McClernan has been a leader in the human potential movement and is currently president of the nonprofit (501-C3) Wellness Institute, International. This organization is devoted to education and research into wellness possibilities. He is considered an authority in health promotion (wellness) and has taught at four universities and a community college.

Currently, Dr. McClernan works for Arrowhead Community Hospital Wellness Center in Phoenix, Arizona. Previously, he worked at the University of Arizona in the Department of Rehabilitation as a research consultant and clinical interviewer.

Dr. McClernan has developed a new health care system he calls "A Cure for Managed Care" and is working with state legislators to set up a demonstration project. This system will give ownership to consumers and to providers, will allow for freedom of choice, and will provide major incentives for members to live healthful lifestyles.